A Practical Guide To Medically Important Fungi and the Diseases They Cause

Alan M. Sugar, M.D.
Evans Memorial Department of Clinical Research and Department of Medicine, Boston Medical Center Boston, Massachusetts Director, Clinical Mycology Center Boston Medical Center

and

Caron A. Lyman, Ph.D.
National Cancer Institute National Institutes of Health Bethesda, Maryland

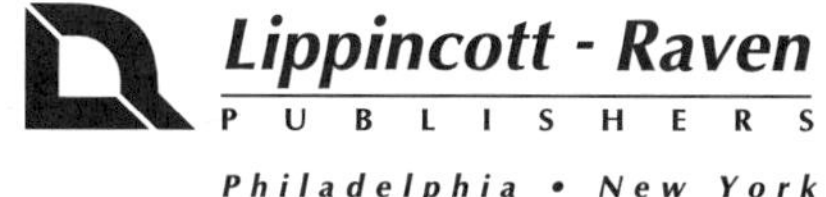
Lippincott - Raven
PUBLISHERS
Philadelphia • New York

Acquisitions Editor: Ruth W. Weinberg
Developmental Editor: Renée Gagliardi
Manufacturing Manager: Dennis Teston
Production Manager: Lawrence Bernstein
Production Editor: Lawrence Bernstein
Cover Designer: Sharon Lewis
Figures: Marilyn Goodlew
Indexer: Susan Lohmeyer
Compositor: Lippincott–Raven Electronic Production
Printer: Maple Press

Printed in the United States of America

9 8 7 6 5 4 3 2 1

Library of Congress Cataloging-in-Publication Data
Sugar, Alan M.
A practical guide to medically important fungi and the diseases they cause / Alan M. Sugar and Caron A. Lyman.
p. cm.
Includes bibliographical references and index.
ISBN 0-397-51686-X
1. Mycoses. 2. Medical mycology I. Lyman, Caron A. I. Title.
[DNLM: 1. Mycoses—microbiology. 2. Mycoses—drug therapy.
3. Fungi—pathogenicity. WC 450 S947p 1997]
RC117.S84 1997
616.9'69—dc21
DNLM/DLC
for Library of Congress

For Carol, Evan, Ian, Glenn, Chris, and Jon
AMS

For Alicia and Melisa, my source of sunshine
CAL

Contents

Part 3–Principles of Antifungal Therapy 95

Appendices 121

Foreword

Now that deep mycoses are no longer a medical curiosity, family practitioners and internists need a readily accessible source of information about diagnosis and treatment of fungal infections. Alan Sugar and Carol Lyman have created a practical book with sufficient detail that the physician can use as a sole source. Practical tables and clear organization make information easy to find. Distinctions between different therapeutic options are lucid. The clinician is told enough of what the diagnostic laboratory does to provide an understanding of the field without providing a flood of unnecessary details. About one fourth of the text is devoted to antifungal agents, including all the current drugs and a little about newer agents under development. The book looks about the right size to fit on a clinician's book shelf, small enough to be handy and big enough to have the necessary information.

John Bennett, M.D.
Head, Clinical Mycology Section
Director, Infectious Diseases Training Program
National Institute of Allergy and Infectious Diseases
National Institutes of Health

Preface

Historically, the fungi have been ignored in the education of physicians because of the infrequency of fungal diseases. When fungal infections were encountered in clinical practice, it resulted in a great deal of consternation. Many practitioners were not familiar with these organisms or the manifestations of fungal disease, and when faced with limited diagnostic and therapeutic options, they felt powerless to be of much assistance to their patients. However, increasing numbers of immunocompromised patients, including those with malignancies, organ transplants, and AIDS, have led to a virtual explosion in the frequency of fungal diseases. Lagging behind, but somewhat parallel with this increase in clinically recognizable mycoses has been the development of the field of antifungal therapeutics. Since amphotericin B was introduced into clinical practice in 1958, no alternative drug was available to treat patients with serious invasive fungal infections. With the introduction of ketoconazole, fluconazole, and itraconazole, and most recently of lipid formulations of amphotericin B, physicians now are faced with choices when deciding on the most appropriate therapeutic option.

While remaining a challenging art, there is a solid foundation upon which to base the diagnosis and treatment of fungal diseases. Many basic principles of infectious diseases apply to fungi and the resultant infections. Moreover, we understand a great deal about the epidemiology and pathogenesis of the more commonly found fungi, knowledge that can be used in the management of our patients. It is a practical, patient-oriented approach that is the focus of this book.

There are comprehensive books that provide detailed information on medical mycology (see Standard Text Sources at the end of this book). However, there has not been a practical, basic, and concise guide to serve as an introduction and a useful companion for those faced with practical questions when confronted with patients with fungal infections. This guide provides easy-to-access, patient-oriented information about the more common fungi and the diseases they cause.

The book is divided into three main sections: Fundamentals of Mycology, The Fungi, and Principles of Antifungal Therapy. Treatment suggestions are provided in the context of the discussion of each infection (Part 2); the particulars of administration of each drug are given in the section devoted to the drugs (Part 3). While the reader may choose a treatment based on the discussion in Part 2, careful consideration should be given to the nuances of patient management in the prescribing of the drug as described in Part 3.

A Practical Guide
To Medically Important Fungi
and the Diseases They Cause

PART 1

Mycology Fundamentals

1

Starting Point: Basics of Medical Mycology

Mycology, the study of the fungi, still remains largely a visual science, even in the era of molecular biology. Certainly, the application of the powerful techniques of molecular biology to problems of identification, diagnosis, and treatment of fungal infections has produced major advances in our understanding of these organisms. However, the routine identification of fungi in the clinical laboratory still depends on careful examination and recognition of the morphology of the organism when it is grown on defined media under defined conditions. Thus, definitive identification of many fungi, especially the molds, may take days or even weeks, depending on the rate of growth and differentiation of the fungus. In this brief introductory chapter, only the basic terminology required to understand the medically important microbiology of these organisms is presented. The interested reader is referred to specialty textbooks for more specific details.

Fungi are eukaryotic organisms and thus share many similarities with animal cells, especially when compared to the prokaryotic bacteria. The major difference between animal and fungal cells is the presence of a rigid cell wall in the fungi. Given their unique position in the world of living things, fungi have been classified in a separate kingdom, Kingdom Fungi, along with the Kingdoms Animals, Plants, and Protists. Thus, the perception that fungi are plants is incorrect, and the ramifications of their eukaryotic physiology are just beginning to be understood with respect to issues concerning pathogenesis and antifungal drug development.

The Kingdom Fungi contains the medically important Classes Ascomycetes, Basidiomycetes, Zygomycetes, and Fungi Imperfecti (Deuteromycetes). Examples of Ascomycetes are *Blastomyces dermatitidis, Histoplasma capsulatum,* and *Aspergillus. Cryptococcus neoformans* is classified as a Basidiomycete, and the Mucorales, such as *Rhizopus, Mucor,* and *Cunninghamella,* are found in the Class Zygomycetes. Clinically important Deuteromycetes include *Candida albicans, Sporothrix schenkii,* and *Coccidioides immitis.* These and many other medically important fungi are discussed in greater depth throughout this text.

Fungi may reproduce by sexual or asexual means; it is through the unique structures of the sexual organisms that classification is often made. The Deuteromycetes are so classified because the perfect or sexual phase has not yet been discovered. This group, therefore, contains many different fungi that are related only by virtue of the lack of an identifiable sexual state. On the other hand, routine identification of fungi depends in large part on the unique morphology of the asexual state of the fungus.

Fungi grow in two basic morphologic forms: yeasts and molds. Yeasts are unicellular structures that reproduce by budding or less commonly by internal subdivision of their cytoplasm. Most often, the mother cell produces only one bud, but multiple buds are found in certain organisms, such as *Paracoccidioides brasiliensis* (see Fig. 8). Adaptations of this basic form have developed and are best illustrated by the spherules of *Coccidioides immitis.* These structures are large (50 to 60 µm in diameter) and reproduce by forming hundreds of smaller endospores within the larger structure (see Fig. 6).

Molds, on the other hand, are multinucleate, and grow in long, filamentous patterns. The filaments, called hyphae, may be subdivided by cross walls, known as septae (as with *Aspergillus*), or they may lack septae (as with the Mucorales). A mass of hyphae is known as mycelia. Specialized hyphae that differentiate into reproductive organs to produce spores (properly termed conidia) are called conidiophores. Much more detailed anatomy of the fungi, as well as a specialized vocabulary, have been developed over the years, but for the nonmycologist, these facts are usually less important than other aspects of the fungi, such as the diseases they cause, their diagnosis, and the best management options available for infected patients.

Some fungi, such as *Candida glabrata,* grow exclusively as yeasts. Others, such as *Aspergillus* and *Fusarium,* grow only as hyphae. Finally, both morphologic forms can be found in different parts of the life cycles of yet other fungi. For example, *C. albicans* can grow in tissue as both yeasts and hyphae. A third form, the pseudohypha, is also formed by this fungus. The distinction is that the appendage arises like a newly formed yeast from budding, with the characteristic stricture between mother and daughter cells, but the newly formed yeast continues to elongate, providing the appearance of the hyphal form. Nutritional factors are most important in the generation of the three different morphologies seen with *C. albicans*. In contrast, the thermally dimorphic fungi grow as hyphae in the environment, but when at the elevated temperatures found in people, they grow solely as yeast-like forms. These fungi include *Blastomyces dermatitidis, Coccidioides immitis, Histoplasma capsulatum, Paracoccidioides brasiliensis,* and *Sporothrix schenkii.* Only in extremely rare situations will the hyphal forms of these fungi be found in human tissues. Fortunately, the yeast-like forms of these fungi are characteristic in appearance so that a presumptive, but usually accurate, diagnosis can be made just by examining microscopic preparations containing the microorganism.

The proper nomenclature for fungi and the diseases they cause is a subject of continuous debate. Matters such as whether the disease caused by *Candida* species should be called candidiasis or candidiosis and whether the invasive infection caused by one of the Mucorales is mucormycosis or zygomycosis continue to appear in the literature. Despite the controversies in nomenclature, fundamental principles and a knowledge base are available to clinicians caring for patients with mycotic infections. It is from this information that this book has been derived.

2

Basic Laboratory Techniques That Can Provide Quick Diagnoses

The clinical signs and symptoms present in patients with fungal infections are often nonspecific and difficult to distinguish from those seen with bacterial infections. Often, antibiotic-resistant fever is the first indication of a fungal infection. While the decision to treat will often be based on the overall clinical picture, it is important to make every effort to isolate and identify the responsible organisms.

Regardless of the expertise of the physician or the microbiologist, the specimen must be properly collected and rapidly transported to the laboratory to increase the likelihood of success in isolating and identifying any organism present. While fungi tend to be less fastidious than viruses and some bacteria, it is important to rapidly process the specimen to minimize the likelihood of overgrowth from rapidly growing, contaminating bacteria.

If a specific fungus is suspected in the differential diagnosis, the laboratory should be notified so that appropriate media may be chosen for culture. In general, specimens sent for fungal culture are inoculated in duplicate onto general mycological isolation media, such as Sabouraud dextrose agar with antibiotics and brain heart infusion agar supplemented with 5% sheep's blood and incubated at 25°C and 35°C. However, most fungi will grow on routine bacteriological isolation media; thus, laboratories processing specimens from immunosuppressed patients should routinely hold their culture plates for up to 4 weeks. When the endemic mycoses are suspected, cultures should be held for 6 weeks.

In addition to culturing, a direct microscopic examination should be performed routinely on all specimens sent to the laboratory. It is important to emphasize that this examination should be done in addition to, not in place of a culture. A 10% KOH solution or calcofluor white may be used to prepare wet mounts. The KOH solution will dissolve most organic material that may be confused with fungi, but without a contrasting dye such as lactophenol cotton blue or blue-black ink, the fungal elements may be difficult to find with an untrained eye. Calcofluor white on the other hand will effectively stain the fungal elements, but a fluorescence microscope is needed. Yeast cells will stain Gram-positive in a routine Gram stain but hyphal elements do not stain uniformly. In peripheral blood smears stained with Wright-Giemsa stain, *Candida* spp. and other yeast will stain dark blue. Histology stains that are not routinely used in the clinical microbiology laboratory should be requested for tissue biopsies. Fungal elements will stain brown to black with methenamine silver stain (GMS), which is useful for detecting low numbers of organisms. Fungal elements also can be seen with routine periodic acid-Schiff (PAS) and less reliably with hematoxylin and eosin (H&E) stained specimens.

BLOOD

The significance of a single blood culture positive for *Candida* spp. has been the topic of much discussion in recent years. As a result of the difficulty in determining in which patients a single positive culture reflects true infection, the relative ease in treating fungemia, and the potentially fatal outcome due to delaying life-saving therapy, treatment is recommended for patients with any blood cultures positive for *Candida* spp. There are a number of detection systems currently available for isolating *Candida* from the bloodstream. These measure variables such as turbidity, infrared signal detection, and production of radioactively labeled CO_2.

While the recovery of *Candida* from the blood has improved with the use of some recently introduced methods, some factors should be kept in mind regardless of the method used. For example, the greater the volume of blood cultured, the greater the likelihood of recovering the invading organism. Venting the blood culture bottles will shorten the time to recovery as well as increase the yield, since *Candida* grow poorly in anaerobic conditions. A biphasic media that combines a solid agar and brain heart infusion (BHI) broth in the same bottle has been reported to further shorten the time to detection of a positive culture. The lysis centrifugation blood culture system has also shortened the time to recovery and increased the sensitivity for detecting not only *Candida* but other fungi, including *Histoplasma capsulatum*, *Cryptococcus neoformans*, as well as some filamentous fungi. This system combines a lysis step with a lytic mixture that destroys the host cells, inactivates complement, and inactivates some antimicrobial agents, with a centrifugation step that concentrates the material that will be cultured.

Cerebrospinal Fluid

The most common fungus encountered in CSF is *Cryptococcus neoformans,* and initial examination of this fluid is directed toward identification of the presence of this yeast-like organism. Diagnosis of cryptococcal meningitis is easily accomplished by the combination of direct examination of the CSF and detection of cryptococcal polysaccharide antigen in CSF. A wet preparation should be examined using India ink to determine if any organisms present in the CSF are encapsulated, suggesting that the fungus is *Cryptococcus neoformans* and not a different organism. A single drop of CSF should be mixed with a single drop of India ink and a cover slip placed on top. Examination of this slide under 400x will reveal round to oval budding yeast cells surrounded by a clear area, which represents the capsule. Occasionally, especially in patients with AIDS, a capsule is not apparent, and then the culture and results of the cryptococcal antigen test will provide helpful adjunctive information.

Tissue Biopsy

As with other specimens, tissue should be processed as soon after collection as possible. It is critical to keep the tissue moist in sterile saline if there will be any delay in transport to the laboratory or in the processing steps after it arrives in the laboratory. If enough sample has been obtained, the tissue should be minced, examined directly in a KOH preparation, and then cultured. The tissue should also be processed in the pathology laboratory so that histopathological examination can also be done.

Examination of Positive Cultures

Cultures should be checked daily or every other day for the presence of growth. Fast growing fungi (e.g., *Candida, Aspergillus*) will appear within 1 to 5 days, while slower-growing fungi (e.g., the dimorphic fungi) may take up to a month to grow. As soon as fungal growth is detected, the organism is subcultured to fresh media to ensure viability.

It is then examined microscopically for budding or sporulation characteristics. If it is too early to make an identification of the fungus, this procedure is repeated until the organism can be identified. Due to the importance of visual characteristics in the identification of fungi, it is important that laboratory personnel note the surface characteristics of the colony, pigmentation on the surface and bottom of the colony (which can diffuse into the agar), the rate of growth, and thermal sensitivity of the fungus. The combination of these features, and in some instances biochemical reactions, will help in the identification of most medically important fungi. In general, simple assimilation and fermentation patterns are used to identify the yeasts, while macroscopic and microscopic appearances are used to identify the majority of molds.

There are a number of methods available for microscopic examination of fungal organisms. While these are reviewed in detail in specialty textbooks and other sources, it is useful to be aware of the existence of these methods. A rapid and useful method is an adhesive tape mount. The sticky side of clear tape is pressed onto the surface of a filamentous colony. While holding the two ends of the tape, it is then gently lifted upward. The tape is then placed on a drop of a blue dye called lactophenol cotton blue (LPCB), which is on the surface of a microscope slide. A cover slip can be applied, and then the slide is examined under a microscope.

From an agar slant, a tease mount may be done. In this case, a small portion of the colony is lifted from the agar with a bent dissecting needle and is placed on a drop of LPCB on a glass slide. With a second dissecting needle, the piece of the fungal colony is teased apart and then covered with a cover slip.

The slowest but best method for determining the details of sporulation and conidiation of a mold is the slide culture. This method is not used if the organism is suspected to be one of the dimorphic fungi, since the geographically restricted dimorphic fungi are highly infectious and need to be handled in a contained environment, such as a biosafety hood. Slide cultures are prepared by placing a small block of sterile agar on a glass slide. The four sides are then inoculated with the specimen. A cover slip is placed on the top of the agar and the slide is placed in a petri dish with moistened filter paper. When the fungus grows, it will grow up onto the cover slip and down onto the glass slide. Once the colony is mature, the glass cover slip is removed and placed into a drop of LPCB on a fresh glass slide and this is then examined under a microscope. The initial slide may also be examined after the agar is removed and a fresh cover slip applied to the area where the fungus is located.

Antifungal Susceptibility Testing

With the increase in number of drugs available to treat invasive mycoses, clinicians now have choices to make when selecting a drug to treat a specific infection. When amphotericin B was the only antifungal drug for almost all of the fungal infections encountered in medicine, there was no need for laboratory testing of any sort. Clearly, the situation has changed, and important decisions need to be made when faced with choosing the most appropriate drug for many different mycoses. Attention has naturally focused on the utility of antifungal susceptibility testing in order to provide the clinician with the necessary information to make an intelligent choice of antifungal drug.

Given the experience with and utility of susceptibility testing of bacteria, it was natural to suspect that similar information could be obtained with fungi. However, due to the differences in physiology between bacteria and fungi, including growth rates, nutritional requirements, temperature requirements, and some unique features of the drugs used to treat patients with mycoses, antifungal susceptibility testing has not been shown to be clinically useful in most situations.

After approximately 15 years of concerted effort, a standardized method for susceptibility testing of yeasts (*Candida* and *Cryptococcus*) has been formulated by participants in several studies sponsored by the National Committee for Clinical Laboratory Standards (NCCLS). What this standardized method has done is to insure reproducibility of results within a given laboratory from day to day and among different laboratories when testing the same isolates. What this method has not done to date is to reliably predict the outcome of therapy of patients with invasive mycoses. It is also important to realize that the current standardized method is not for testing molds.

Several modifications of the NCCLS standardized broth dilution tests have been proposed, including modifications to the composition of the media and, most importantly, adapting microtiter plate testing methodology to replace the large test tubes specified in the standard method. This microtiter method is easily adaptable for the routine hospital microbiology laboratory, but since the meaning of the results is often not clear, interpretation of the data by experts is invaluable. (Some laboratories important in the development of standard susceptibility testing methods and ability to function as reference laboratories are listed in Appendix 20.)

The one potential clinical use for susceptibility testing is in AIDS patients with thrush who have disease that resists treatment with fluconazole. The usual clinical setting is an AIDS patient with a very low CD4 count and thrush not responding to fluconazole (200 to 400 mg daily). *Candida albicans* is usually implicated, but non-albicans species are also recovered. When tested using the NCCLS method, the MICs of these isolates will typically be >32 μg/ml, whereas MICs from *Candida* responding to these doses of fluconazole typically are <8 μg/ml. Resistance may extend to other azoles, such as itraconazole and ketoconazole, but not always, so testing against these drugs should also be performed. Choice of the most appropriate treatment strategy in this situation is discussed in Chapter 4.

PART 2

The Fungi

INTRODUCTION TO THE FUNGI

More than 200,000 species of fungi have been characterized. However, only about 200 of these have been recognized as pathogenic. The fungi discussed in the coming pages are divided, somewhat artificially, into the "opportunistic" fungi and the "dimorphic" fungi. The opportunistic fungi are those that usually cause disease in people who have an abnormal immune system and who cannot fend off these otherwise relatively avirulent microorganisms. Given that the degree of immunosuppression and the number of immunosuppressed patients are increasing at an unprecedented pace, fungi previously thought to be nonpathogenic are being recovered from patients with unusual infections. Thus, these so-called saprophytic fungi are capable of causing disease given a suitable host. Opportunistic fungi usually do not cause serious infections in the immunocompetent host.

In contrast, the dimorphic fungi are capable of causing disease in immunocompetent people. The most important point to remember is that any fungus can infect as an opportunist in a suitably immunocompromised host. Thus, any fungus recovered from a patient needs to be identified, and correlation of the clinical and microbiological results is always necessary. Consultation with experts in dealing with diagnosis and management issues will often be necessary and helpful. Interaction with reference laboratories (listed on page 142) may also help with choosing appropriate diagnostic and therapeutic laboratory tests and with their interpretation.

THE "OPPORTUNISTIC" FUNGI

The opportunistic fungi usually do not cause invasive disease, since a normal immune system keeps these fungi from growing, even after they have entered the body (usually the lungs). For example, spores of *Aspergillus* species and *Rhizopus* species are ubiquitous—and humans inhale conidia (spores) from these organisms virtually every day. While many spores are the appropriate size for easy entry into the alveoli (2 to 5 µm), clinically evident infection almost never follows their inhalation.

The spores remain dormant in the airways and lungs, and are eventually cleared in people with normal immune systems. In contrast, however, such spores can cause life-threatening infection in patients with abnormalities in their immune system. The important message is that virtually any fungus can cause disease if exposure and immunocompromise are optimal. Therefore, any patient who is immunosuppressed by underlying disease or drugs is at risk for the development of an invasive fungal infection. Any yeast or mold recovered from such patients should not be dismissed as a "contaminant" or colonizer without first ruling out its role in the pathogenesis of the patient's condition.

Many risk factors predispose a person to the development of an invasive fungal infection. The primary defect in many patients seems to be neutrophil-related, especially chemotherapy-induced neutropenia. Patients who undergo cytotoxic chemotherapy often have marrow aplasia, and during their course of neutropenia, the risk of developing fungal infections increases exponentially with time. Persistent fever for more than 4 to 7 days while neutropenic patients are receiving broad spectrum antibacterial agents very often is due to early invasive mycosis. Institution of amphotericin B at this time results in defervescence and decreased morbidity. Depressed cell-mediated immunity, such as occurs with high-dose corticosteroid therapy, also results in enhanced risk of developing systemic mycoses, but these are typically different than those associated with neutropenia.

TABLE 1. *Risk Factors and Fungi Commonly Associated with Them*

Predisposing Host Factors	Fungi
Neutropenia	*Aspergillus* *Candida* (hematogenous, disseminated) agents of mucormycosis *Fusarium* other molds
Cell-mediated immune deficits (including AIDS)	*Candida* (mucosal) *Cryptococcus*
Malnutrition	agents of mucormycosis *Aspergillus* *Trichosporon*
Diabetes mellitus	agents of mucormycosis *Candida* (mucosal)
Steroids	*Cryptococcus* *Candida* agents of mucormycosis
Cytotoxic chemotherapy	*Aspergillus* *Candida*

The predisposing risk factors and the fungi most often associated with specific factors are summarized in Table 1. A differential diagnosis of the fungi most likely to be the cause of infection can often be narrowed just on the basis of understanding the immune defect present in a given patient.

3

Aspergillus

Aspergillus species are responsible for a wide range of clinically important manifestations. The spectrum of diseases include saprophytic colonization, allergic manifestations, superficial mucosal infections, and invasive, tissue-destructive infections (Table 2). While the genus *Aspergillus* includes more than 600 species, only a handful have been implicated in causing human infection. The three most commonly isolated species of *Aspergillus* involved in human disease are *A. fumigatus, A. flavus,* and *A. niger.* The more severely immunocompromised the patient, the more likely that the recovery of the fungus will be associated with manifestations of tissue invasion and the need for aggressive

TABLE 2. *Diseases Caused By Aspergillus*

Allergic type diseases
Asthma
Allergic bronchopulmonary aspergillosis (ABPA)
Fungus ball (mycetoma)
Invasive diseases
<u>Acute</u>
Pulmonary
pneumonia
lung abscess
tracheobronchitis
Paranasal sinusitis
Endocarditis
Eye
keratomycosis
endophthalmitis
Cutaneous
Gastrointestinal
<u>Chronic</u>
Chronic necrotizing pulmonary aspergillosis

medical or surgical management. Thus, determination of the significance of a positive culture for *Aspergillus* is highly dependent on the clinical status of the patient and the species isolated.

ALLERGIC BRONCHIAL ASTHMA

Clinical

Sensitization to *Aspergillus* antigens can occur in asthmatic patients, possibly secondary to the trapping of *Aspergillus* conidia in the thick secretions characteristically seen in these patients. Patients are typically atopic and this hypersensitivity reaction can precipitate and perpetuate bronchospasm.

Diagnosis

Elevation of eosinophils and total IgE are often present. Specific IgE responses to *Aspergillus* can also be demonstrated in these patients. Otherwise, the condition presents clinically as typical asthma.

Treatment

No specific antifungal treatment is indicated in these patients, other than an attempt to decrease exposure to *Aspergillus* conidia, a difficult, if not impossible, task. Usual treatment for asthma is all that is required.

ALLERGIC BRONCHOPULMONARY ASPERGILLOSIS (ABPA)

Clinical

This condition is a syndrome based on a host allergic response to the presence of *Aspergillus* antigens. *A. fumigatus* is the most common species involved, but *A. flavus, A. terreus,* and *A. niger* also have been recovered from patients with ABPA. Tissue invasion does not occur and symptoms develop as a result of hypersensitivity to the fungus. In addition to bronchospasm, patients with ABPA often experience the expectoration of brown mucous plugs containing *Aspergillus* and eosinophils.

On occasion, other fungi, such as *Rhizopus,* have resulted in a similar clinical condition. Steroid-responsive asthma and cystic fibrosis are two common underlying conditions in patients with this diagnosis.

Diagnosis

Eight criteria have been suggested as indicative of ABPA:

- Episodic wheezing (asthma)
- Eosinophilia
- Immediate skin test reactivity to *Aspergillus* antigens
- Precipitating (IgG) antibodies to *Aspergillus*
- Elevated total IgE
- Elevated *Aspergillus*-specific IgE
- Central bronchiectasis
- History of pulmonary infiltrates

The diagnosis of ABPA should be considered in the differential diagnosis in patients with asthma, eosinophilia, and a history of unexplained pulmonary infiltrates. Patients meeting at least seven of the above criteria have a high likelihood of having ABPA and the presence of all eight of the criteria make the diagnosis certain. Once the diagnosis is established, steroids should be instituted in an attempt to control bronchospasm and decrease the likelihood of developing permanent structural changes in the lungs, such as bronchiectasis.

Treatment

Treatment of ABPA usually requires the use of prednisone, 0.5 mg/kg/day for approximately 2 weeks. The steroids can then be given on alternate days for about 3 months. Tapering the dose, with attention to symptoms, can then be attempted at a rate of 5 mg every 2 weeks. Response to therapy can be assessed by noting improvement of symptoms in the chest x-ray and a decrease in total serum IgE concentrations. Studies suggest that adjunctive therapy with itraconazole (200 mg, given orally twice daily) may be beneficial by reducing the total antigen burden of the patient. Insufficient information concerning duration of itraconazole treatment is available, but months of therapy probably will be needed if this drug is used.

FUNGUS BALL

Clinical

Aspergillus species may infect previously established cavities in the lungs, with the formation of a mass of hyphae, known as a fungus ball or mycetoma. Patients with previous tuberculosis, sarcoidosis, or prior invasive aspergillosis are most likely to suffer from this disease, since the resultant cavities can be colonized with *Aspergillus*. Patients with fungus balls often are asymptomatic, but with time, most develop some manifestation of illness. Cough and hemoptysis are the most common symptoms; fever and weight loss occur much less frequently. Secondary bacterial infection of *Aspergillus*-filled cavities also can occur, producing signs and symptoms of acute infection.

Approximately 10% of patients with fungus balls have spontaneous resolution of the problem. Most patients will suffer from at least one episode of hemoptysis and massive hemoptysis may occur in up to 20% of patients. The risk of this latter complication increases with the duration of the disease.

Diagnosis

While sputum cultures may be positive for the fungus, many patients with fungus balls have repeatedly negative cultures. Serum anti-*Aspergillus* IgG titers may be increased, but skin testing is not recommended. On chest x-ray, a cavity containing a mass should be visualized. Surrounding the mass may be a crescent of air, giving rise to a typical "crescent halo" (Monod's sign). The intracavitary mass may be mobile and can be demonstrated in patients who have x-rays done while they are in various positions. Chest computed tomography (CT) scans are also useful in evaluating the periphery of the cavity and can detect possible tissue-invasive activity surrounding the cavity. Many patients with such invasive disease are given the additional diagnosis of chronic invasive aspergillosis (see below) and require additional specific antifungal therapy.

Treatment

Treatment for *Aspergillus* fungus balls is dependent on the severity of symptoms and the presence of chronic lung disease. If hemoptysis or other manifestations of the infection are troublesome, itraconazole, 200 mg bid, has been used and may be effective. Similarly, if there is a contraindication to oral therapy with itraconazole, intravenous amphotericin B, 0.6 to 1.0 mg/kg/day, can be used. More frequent episodes of hemoptysis or large amounts of bleeding are indications for surgical evaluation for extirpation of the cavity. However, some patients may not be surgical candidates because of their underlying pulmonary disease. A coordinated approach between infectious disease and pulmonary physicians and thoracic surgeons is needed to accomplish the maximum benefit for each patient. Bacterial superinfections should be treated with appropriate antibacterial antibiotics.

INVASIVE ASPERGILLOSIS

Virtually any organ of the body can be involved with infection due to *Aspergillus* species. However, the respiratory tract is the most commonly affected area, and certain clinical presentations routinely occur with this fungal infection. Amphotericin B remains the mainstay of therapy for most cases of invasive aspergillosis, although some alternatives are discussed below.

Acute Syndromes

The more common invasive syndromes are acute conditions, and occur in patients with immunocompromise, especially neutropenia. The exact clinical presentation depends on the location of the infection. Being an airborne organism, most patients will have involvement of the respiratory tract. Sinusitis, with features similar to those of mucormycosis, is being increasingly recognized. Invasive pneumonitis is also an emerging problem in the neutropenic patient. Patients with apparently isolated brain, liver, or other organ involvement most likely had an initial asymptomatic phase of respiratory tract disease. One exception to this is the rare patient with disseminated or isolated nonpulmonary organ aspergillosis who acquired the infection during the injection of illicit drugs, in a manner similar to the intravenous drug user (IVDU) who develops mucormycosis.

Pneumonia

Clinical

This manifestation of aspergillosis occurs primarily in the patient who is rendered neutropenic by chemotherapy. Children with chronic granulomatous disease as well as patients with end stage AIDS also may develop invasive pulmonary aspergillosis. The common predisposition, however, is a quantitative or qualitative abnormality of the neutrophil. As with all forms of invasive aspergillosis, tissue invasion with a predilection for blood vessels is routinely seen. The infection can progress rapidly with significant amounts of lung necrosis developing over several days. Alternatively, some patients may have enough host response to slow the progression of disease over several weeks. In these patients, cavitary lesions may develop and a fungus ball composed of *Aspergillus* hyphae may appear. Patients usually will have fever and may complain of chest pain, hemoptysis, and dyspnea. Untreated, this infection may disseminate from the lungs, and infection of other organs can then occur. Manifestations of infection of these nonpulmonary sites may dominate the clinical picture.

Diagnosis

Isolation of an *Aspergillus* spp. from expectorated pulmonary secretions collected from a febrile neutropenic patient with pulmonary infiltrates provides strong evidence of pulmonary aspergillosis. However, culture of the fungus from secretions is not necessary for presumptive diagnosis of aspergillosis in the suitably predisposed host. In this case, pulmonary symptoms, a compatible chest x-ray and the presence of neutropenia, corticosteroid use or other immunosuppression is enough to warrant the institution of amphotericin B. The chest x-ray may show manifestations such as bronchopneumonia, segmental pneumonia, lobar consolidation, nodular lesions, or cavitary lesions. CT scans may reveal lesions not yet apparent on chest x-ray, such as crescentic cavitary lesions. Since most patients at risk for *Aspergillus* pneumonia have thrombocytopenia in addition to their neutrophil defect, invasive procedures for diagnostic purposes, such as bronchoscopy, may not be feasible, and therapy must be instituted for presumed infection. This is one of the scenarios supporting the empiric use of amphotericin B in the persistently febrile neutropenic patient.

Treatment

In the critically ill patient, amphotericin B is used (1 to 1.5 mg/kg/day). As more experience with liposomal formulations of amphotericin B become available, these may replace conventional amphotericin B as first-line therapy. In patients who are not critically ill and who can take oral medication, itraconazole, 200 mg bid, can be used, but serum concentrations of the drug should be monitored to insure that the drug is being absorbed. Duration of therapy is dictated in large part by the response of the infection, but many months may be needed to effect a cure. Resolution of the neutropenia and minimization of other immunosuppressive medications is critical to the success of therapy. Failure of the bone marrow to recover in the neutropenic patient dooms antifungal therapy. The use of cytokines, such as granulocyte colony stimulating factor (G-CSF) or granulocyte/macrophage colony stimulating factor (GM-CSF), as adjunctive antifungal agents is still experimental but may work by increasing the number of neutrophils as well as enhancing function of existing phagocytic cells. Given the high cost and uncertain benefits of this therapy, cytokines cannot be routinely recommended for use in this patient population at this time.

Disseminated Aspergillosis

Clinical

Dissemination of infection follows clinically apparent or unnoticed pulmonary infection. Patients are usually severely immunocompromised with absent neutrophils or other critical abnormalities of their immune systems. Infection of virtually any organ can occur with symptoms referable to the area of infection. Fever and signs of overwhelming infection, such as hypotension, altered mental status, and renal and hepatic dysfunction may be present. Interestingly, cutaneous manifestations of infection are lacking, in contrast to patients with disseminated fusariosis, who often have skin lesions. However, since *Aspergillus* spp. invade blood vessels, superficial necrosis secondary to thromboembolism of the superficial blood supply can occur.

Diagnosis

Recovery of the fungus from biopsy specimens obtained from clinically infected areas is definitive. Presumptive diagnosis of disseminated aspergillosis is made when septate hyphae are visualized under the microscope, but not yet grown in the laboratory.

Treatment

Amphotericin B is the mainstay of therapy in these patients, since oral therapy is not usually feasible, given the critical condition of the patients. Higher doses are used initially (1.0 to 1.5 mg/kg/day) to stabilize the patient. After days to weeks, if oral therapy is possible, a switch to itraconazole, 200 mg bid, can be considered. Duration of therapy is dependent upon the degree and persistence of immunosuppression, but typically lasts for at least several months.

Lung Abscess

Clinical

The natural history of invasive pulmonary aspergillosis may include the development of one or more cavities as a result of tissue necrosis. Typically cavitation occurs as the neutrophil count recovers in patients who had a prior episode of neutropenia. Patients may be febrile and develop chest pain, cough, and hemoptysis. Fever, malaise, and fatigue are often common complaints.

Diagnosis

Culture of expectorated sputum may yield *Aspergillus* species, but many patients do not produce sputum. The differential diagnosis of a cavitary lesion is quite broad, including pyogenic bacteria, *Nocardia, Actinomyces,* fungi, occasionally viruses, and noninfectious causes such as malignancies, collagen vascular diseases, and pulmonary embolism. Thus, aspiration of the contents of the cavity or biopsy of the cavity wall through a bronchoscope or via a percutaneous route may be required in order to select the most appropriate therapy. Narrow, septate hyphae with acute angle branching compatible with *Aspergillus* spp. are typically seen (Fig. 1) on KOH preparation of the biopsy material, and cultures may grow the fungus within several weeks.

Treatment

Therapy for 3 to 6 months or more is usually required. If the patient can tolerate itraconazole, this is a good choice for such long-term therapy. Doses of 200 mg twice daily are usually used. If the patient is extremely ill, amphotericin B can be used initially; and the switch to itraconazole can be made once the patient is stabilized. Surgery may be warranted for patients with severe hemoptysis. Secondary bacterial

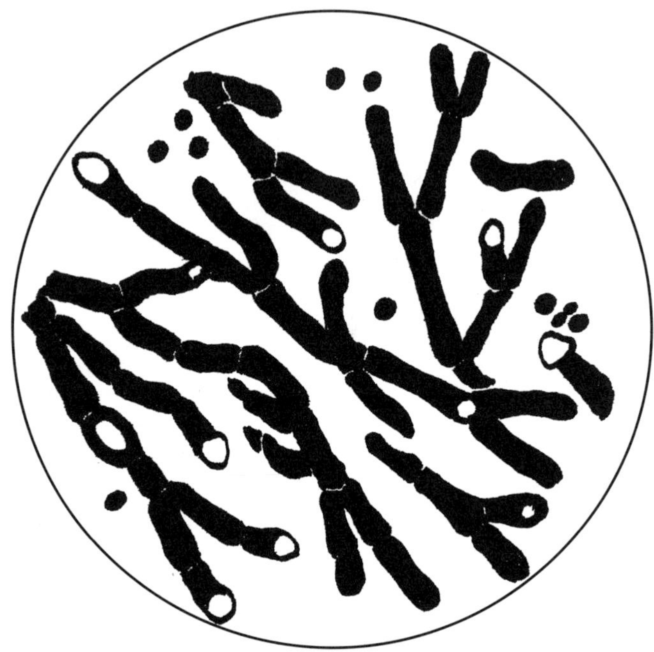

FIG. 1. Narrow, septate hyphae with acute angle branching, suggestive of *Aspergillus, Fusarium,* and *Pseudallescheria boydii* (*Scedosporium*).

infection of the cavitary lesion should be treated with appropriate antibacterial antibiotics.

Tracheobronchitis

Clinical

This is a relatively recently recognized manifestation of aspergillosis occurring primarily in patients with AIDS, but also has been described in patients with lung transplants and those with neutropenia. In the latter group of patients, however, tracheobronchitis most often is associated with invasive lung involvement. The disease is characterized by circumferential infection of the airways with the formation of pseudomembranes. As these enlarge, plugging of the airways can follow, with resulting atelectasis of the pulmonary parenchyma and postobstructive pneumonia. Patients complain primarily of dyspnea and other signs and symptoms may include low-grade fever, cough, and expectoration of the plugs.

Diagnosis

The chest x-ray may be normal, but areas of atelectasis involving lung distal to the airway process can be seen. Cultures of sputum will usually be positive for *Aspergillus* species (usually *A. fumigatus*). If a plug can be examined it is packed with *Aspergillus* hyphae. Bronchoscopy, with biopsy of the mucosal plaques, may be required to secure a definitive diagnosis.

Treatment

Itraconazole has been reported to be useful in the treatment of this infection. Doses of 200 mg twice daily are usually sufficient. Alternatively, amphotericin B, 0.6 to 1.0 mg/kg/day, can be used for initial therapy, or for the full course of therapy, which may last several months, depending on the response to treatment and the presence and degree of the underlying condition.

Sinusitis

Clinical

Aspergillus spp. also may be involved in infections of the upper airways, and a disease indistinguishable from mucormycosis may ensue. It can occur prior to or concomitantly with pulmonary aspergillosis. Patients may present with nasal congestion, fever, or facial pain. Extension of the disease from the sinuses to the orbit will result in eye pain, blurred vision, proptosis, or chemosis, depending on the location of the infectious process. Extension posteriorly into the brain can result in mental status changes, lethargy, or seizures.

Diagnosis

Definitive diagnosis is dependent on identification of the fungus in tissue biopsies of nasal septal lesions or sinus aspirates. However, since many of these patients are thrombocytopenic, biopsies may not be feasible. Thus, microscopic visualization or culture of an *Aspergillus* spp. from superficial swabs or nasal discharge collected from high-risk neutropenic patients can be taken as presumptive evidence of aspergillosis. X-rays of the paranasal sinuses may reveal sinus opacification, while

CT or magnetic resonance imaging (MRI) may reveal mucosal thickening, bone destruction, or air-fluid levels. Involvement of the areas surrounding the sinuses also may be demonstrable on the scans.

Treatment

As with pneumonia caused by *Aspergillus* spp., amphotericin B is the mainstay of therapy for *Aspergillus* sinusitis in the critically ill patient (described above). Itraconazole, 200 mg bid, also may be useful in selected cases, especially when long-term therapy is required to cure the infection. Since sinuses and structures in the face are more accessible to more accurate diagnosis and surgical intervention, aggressive debridement of devitalized tissue should complement medical management of these patients.

Endocarditis

Clinical

Endocarditis caused by *Aspergillus* spp. is a rare infection occurring almost exclusively on prosthetic valves. Blood cultures are rarely positive, and the diagnosis is made on the basis of identification of the fungus in an embolus to a large artery or examination of the infected valve at surgery. Hemodynamic instability may occur as a result of large, bulky vegetations on the valve and manifestations of valvular insufficiency or stenosis can be seen. Embolic phenomena will lead to site-specific symptoms, depending on the location of the clot.

Diagnosis

Echocardiography may aid in the demonstration of the vegetations and other cardiac pathology. Histopathologic examination of a clot or the vegetation will reveal the presence of narrow, regular, acute, angle-branched septate hyphae. This picture is consistent with the presence of *Aspergillus* spp., but *Fusarium* spp., *Pseudallescheria* spp., and other molds must also be considered. Definitive diagnosis is established when the fungus grows from a culture of the clot or vegetation, which could take from days to several weeks. However, *Aspergillus* spp. normally grow within 5 days.

Treatment

Treatment of this manifestation of aspergillosis often requires surgical replacement of the involved valve in addition to therapy with amphotericin B, in initial doses of 1 to 1.5 mg/kg/day. Subsequently, amphotericin B can be decreased to 0.8 to 1 mg/kg/day if the patient can tolerate this dosage. Should this dose of conventional amphotericin B not be tolerated by the patient, a liposomal formulation of amphotericin B may represent a useful alternative. The role of itraconazole is not known, but it seems reasonable to consider a course of life-long suppression with oral itraconazole, 200 mg once or twice daily, given the propensity of this infection to recur once medical therapy is stopped.

Eye

Both anterior and posterior segments of the eye may become infected with *Aspergillus* spp. The disease may be secondary to trauma with direct implantation of the fungus, or be the result of dissemination from a distant, usually pulmonary, focus.

Keratitis

Clinical

Trauma to the eye may be complicated by the development of *Aspergillus* infection. Initially, involvement of the cornea will occur, but deeper structures may be affected as a complete endophthalmitis evolves. Patients with keratitis present with redness and pain, due to ulceration of the cornea. Visual acuity may be decreased. Patients may complain of photophobia and/or excessive tearing. Keratitis may be caused by a variety of microorganisms, making a specific etiologic diagnosis possible only after the organism is identified in the laboratory. In fact, most patients with fungal keratitis will have been treated for bacterial or viral keratitis before fungi are suspected.

Diagnosis

The first step in making the diagnosis is considering the presence of a fungus in the differential. Since the organism is present in the corneal stroma, simple swabbing of the surface of the cornea is insufficient to recover *Aspergillus* spp. Corneal scrapings do, however, provide the material needed for recovery of the organism. These scrapings should be examined microscopically as well as cultured on specific media to encourage growth of fungi and to inhibit bacterial growth (see Chapter 2). Direct microscopic examination of scrapings often reveal hyphal elements, which is important for making a timely diagnosis.

Treatment

Topical therapy with a polyene, such as natamycin (5% solution) has been used with some success in treating this infection; clotrimazole (1% solution) can also be used. Should systemic therapy be desired, itraconazole (200 mg twice daily) or amphotericin B (0.6 to 1.0 mg/kg/day) can be used in addition to the topical therapy.

Endophthalmitis

Clinical

Aspergillus spp. can reach the eye through hematogenous spread or by direct inoculation, such as following trauma or surgery on the eye. Spread through the circulation it is usually found in patients with *Aspergillus* endocarditis or in intravenous drug abusers. Occasionally, patients with abnormal immune systems also will have endophthalmitis as part of disseminated aspergillosis. Patients may present with eye pain, erythema, or blurred vision. Examination of the eye may show involvement of all of the structures in the orbit, and lesions can be seen on direct visualization of the retina. Retinal hemorrhages and hypopyon may occur. Proptosis, retinal detachment, or erosion of the sclera also may occur as the disease progresses.

Diagnosis

The presentation is compatible with other infectious causes of endophthalmitis, and diagnosis is dependent on the recovery of the fungus from suitable specimens. If the cornea is involved, scrapings may contain the typical acute angle branching hyphae of *Aspergillus* spp. Aspiration of the anterior chamber or of the vitreous also may be useful in that the hyphae may be present on microscopic examination or culture of this material. The fungal elements typically surround blood vessels.

Treatment

Therapy includes treatment of the eye infection as well as any other involved site. Intravenous amphotericin B has been the mainstay of the medical management in patients with *Aspergillus* endophthalmitis. The usual dose will be approximately 1 mg/kg/day. In addition, low doses of amphotericin B (e.g., 10 μg) may be injected directly into the vitreous, and subconjunctival injections of 200 μg also can be used to supplement the intravenous regimen. While theoretically appealing, use of itraconazole has been very limited in treating patients with *Aspergillus* endophthalmitis. Thus, firm recommendations concerning its role in therapy cannot be made. Consultation with an ophthalmologist and an experienced infectious diseases specialist is strongly encouraged. Reversal of any underlying predisposing factors, if possible, is also desirable.

Cutaneous Aspergillosis

Clinical

Cutaneous manifestations of aspergillosis occur usually as a result of direct implantation of the organism into the skin. Predisposing factors include trauma and prior surgery. Less commonly, this fungus spreads hematogenously from other organs to involve the skin. Patients usually present with ulcerated lesions, which may progress rapidly or more slowly, depending on the degree of underlying immunosuppression.

Diagnosis

Definitive diagnosis depends on the results from a biopsy of the lesion. The dichotomously branching, septate hyphae, typically seen microscopically, are most easily recognized on tissue sections stained with Gomori methenamine silver (GMS) or periodic acid Schiff (PAS). With careful examination, they may also be seen on routine hematoxylin and eosin (H&E) stained sections (Fig. 1). The organism may grow in culture of the biopsy specimen within several days, but cultures should be held for at least 4 weeks before being signed out as negative.

Treatment

Amphotericin B has been the mainstay of therapy. Doses in the range of 0.6 to 1.5 mg/kg/day are usually more effective than lower amounts in the treatment of aspergillosis, but the status of predisposing factors and severity of the infection are important correlates of prognosis. Higher doses should be used in more critically ill patients. However, in patients who can tolerate oral therapy and who are not critically ill, itraconazole, 200 mg bid, is a reasonable alternative.

Gastrointestinal Disease

Clinical

Gastrointestinal disease is a rare manifestation of aspergillosis, usually a result of severe immunocompromise, especially prolonged and profound neutropenia. Patients may present with symptoms and signs of an acute abdomen, with pain, rigidity, and few to no bowel sounds. Diarrhea may be present. Fever also usually occurs.

Diagnosis

This diagnosis is usually made postmortem, since the infection typically occurs in critically ill patients with advanced primary diseases. Moreover, the diagnosis is difficult to make, since isolation or visualization of the fungus is needed. Positive culture or presence of typical hyphae on microscopic examination of biopsy material warrants institution of therapy and evaluation of the patient for the presence of *Aspergillus* in other areas of the body.

Treatment

Amphotericin B is the treatment of choice in doses of 1 to 1.5 mg/kg/day. This can be reduced to 0.8 to 1.0 mg/kg/day if the patient improves and as dictated by toxicity. Liposomal formulations of amphotericin B may also be used, but experience with these formulations for this unusual indication is very limited. Similarly, once the patient has been stabilized and the infection is brought under some control, consideration can be given to the use of itraconazole. However, since this azole must be given orally, good conditions must exist for oral absorption of the drug, i.e., acid pH, food in stomach (see Chapter 17).

Chronic Syndromes

Clinical

Chronic invasive aspergillosis is a term given to an indolent infection of the lungs, sometimes associated with pulmonary fungus balls. The infection is present for weeks to months and may be associated with low-grade fevers, weight loss, and hemoptysis. This condition may represent one stage in the continuum from saprophytic colonization to acute pneumonitis.

Diagnosis

The chest x-ray in patients with chronic pulmonary aspergillosis will show slowly evolving infiltrates, often patchy and associated with concomitant underlying pulmonary disease. CT scans may be more sensitive in identifying areas of necrotic lung, blood vessel invasion, and consolidation than are conventional chest x-rays.

Treatment

Since this is an indolent infection and patients are not usually critically ill, itraconazole, 200 mg bid, is a good choice for initial therapy. Serum concentrations should be monitored, and attention should be given to potential drug interactions. Hemoptysis may require surgical intervention; or if the source of bleeding can be localized, embolization of the bleeding artery can be attempted.

4

Candida

The spectrum of disease caused by *Candida* is extensive. The range of manifestations extends from simple mucosal colonization to multiple organ invasion (Table 3). The most common mucosal surfaces involved are the mouth, vagina, and esophagus. Bladder infection with *Candida* also can be considered a mucosal infection. Candidiasis occurs in all age groups, from diaper rash or invasive candidiasis in the neonate through mucosal or invasive disease in the elderly. While it is known that neutrophils are important in host defense against the development of organ invasion and that cell-mediated immunity (i.e., T lymphocytes and macrophages) is an important defender of the mucosae, many of the specific details of the interactions between yeasts and the human immune system remain unresolved. However, patients with neutropenia, such as bone marrow transplant recipients or leukemics who receive cytotoxic chemotherapy, are at increased risk of developing candidemia, hepatosplenic candidiasis, and other serious invasive manifestations of candidiasis. In contrast, those with cell-mediated immune deficits, such as AIDS patients, most often present with evidence of mucosal candidiasis. In fact, the development of thrush in HIV-infected patients often indicates a drop in the CD4 lymphocyte count to 200/mm^3 or less.

Members of the genus *Candida* have been increasingly recovered from patients with serious infections. The most common species encountered in clinical practice include *C. albicans, C. tropicalis, C. parapsilosis, C. glabrata* (*Torulopsis glabrata*), and *C. krusei*. It is important to identify the species of *Candida* isolated because of different patterns of drug susceptibility. Species other than those listed also may be recovered from patients and should not be ignored as clinically unimportant (e.g., *C. lusitaniae, C. rugosa, C. pseudotropicalis, C. guillermondii,* and others).

TABLE 3. *Manifestations of Infection Due to Candida*

Superficial candidiasis
Oropharyngeal candidiasis (thrush)
Vulvovaginitis
Cutaneous infection, including diaper rash, tinea
Chronic mucocutaneous candidiasis
Onychomycosis
Invasive candidiasis
Localized
Esophagitis
Gastrointestinal
Urinary tract—cystitis, fungus balls, localized renal infection
Peritonitis—including that secondary to perforated viscus and CAPD
Hematogenously disseminated candidiasis
Candidemia—may be associated with multiple organ involvement, including eye, bones, skin, heart, kidney, etc.
Chronic disseminated candidiasis (hepatosplenic candidiasis)
Suppurative thrombophlebitis
Endophthalmitis
Osteomyelitis
Endocarditis
Myocardium
Arthritis
Meningitis
Brain abscess
Pneumonia (very rare)

CAPD = Continuous ambulatory peritoneal dialysis

SUPERFICIAL CANDIDIASIS

Oropharyngeal candidiasis

Clinical

This common mucosal condition is found primarily in immunocompromised patients, but also may occur in patients who are treated with antibiotics (Table 4). There are several different presentations of infection of the mouth and throat with *Candida* (Table 5). Thrush (pseudomembranous candidiasis) is the most common oral manifestation, char-

TABLE 4. *Patients at Risk for Thrush*

Cancer chemotherapy
Radiation therapy of the head and neck
AIDS
Inhaled corticosteroids

TABLE 5. *Manifestations of Oropharyngeal Candidiasis*

Thrush
Atrophic candidiasis [acute and chronic (denture-related)]
Angular cheilitis
Leukoplakia

acteristically identified by the thick white patches on the tongue, buccal mucosa, hard palate, and gingivae. These patches are comprised of yeast, desquamated epithelial cells, white blood cells, debris, and bacteria. The underlying mucosal surface is often inflamed, and may bleed when the patches are removed. The fungi are readily identified by placing this white material on a slide with 10% KOH, which disrupts all of the host cellular components and debris without lysing the fungi.

Acute atrophic candidiasis presents with atrophy of the tongue, and can be a sequela of acute episodes of thrush. Chronic atrophic candidiasis is predominantly a disease related to *Candida*-infected dentures. Both patient and dentures need to be treated to avoid repeated inoculation of the palate.

Angular cheilitis presents with cracks at the corners of the mouth and can be caused by bacteria as well as *Candida*. An inflammatory reaction to the infection is thought to result in skin breakdown in this highly mobile area of the anatomy.

Candida leukoplakia is characterized by the presence of hard white plaques on the lips, buccal mucosa, and tongue. These lesions are distinct from the curd-like patches of thrush and may be premalignant.

Diagnosis

Diagnosis is often apparent from the clinical appearance of the mucosal lesions. However, in granulocytopenic patients, apparent thrush actually may be due to Herpes simplex virus or mixed bacterial flora. Therefore, visualization of the fungus under the microscope and identification of the microorganism in the microbiology laboratory are important to confirm the diagnosis and to help direct therapy. A sample of the lesion can be scraped with a tongue depressor and placed on a glass microscope slide with a drop of 10% KOH. After a cover slip is placed on the preparation, the yeast, pseudohyphae, and hyphae may be seen at 400x power (Fig. 2). A sample of the lesion should be obtained on a sterile cotton swab following vigorous scraping of the oral lesion and sent to the laboratory for culture.

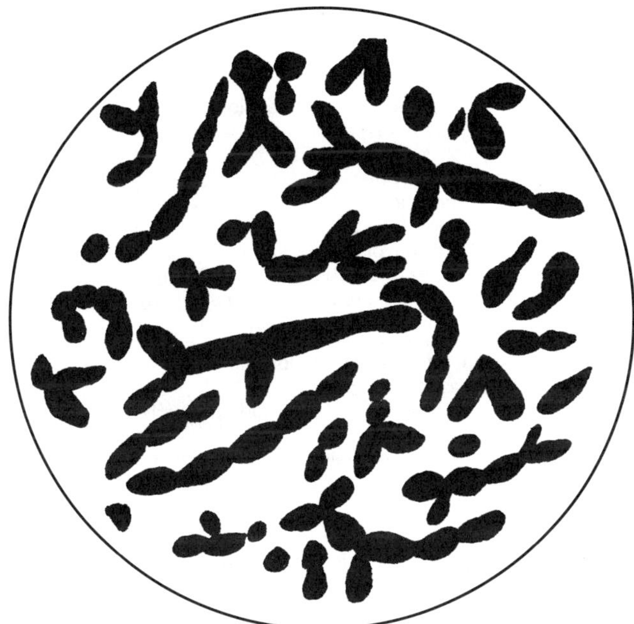

FIG. 2. Budding yeasts, pseudohyphae, and hyphae suggestive of *Candida albicans.* True hyphae are not formed by most other Candida species, but pseudohyphae can be seen in tissue.

Treatment

There are many different preparations available for the treatment of thrush and other manifestations of oral candidiasis (Table 6). In patients without chronic predisposing factors, treatment can range from 5 to 14 days, with good responses evident within several days of starting treatment. In these patients, little evidence suggests superiority of one drug or formulation over another. However, while initial responses to therapy may be good in patients with persistent underlying predisposing conditions, such as malignancy or AIDS, relapse of the infection often occurs. In AIDS patients, fluconazole has been shown to be superior to topical treatment with nystatin suspension, both clinically and mycologically, based on its ability to eradicate the fungi.

Recently, resistance to fluconazole has been noted in AIDS patients who typically receive the drug for prolonged periods. AIDS patients often are treated for the first episodes of thrush with lower doses of fluconazole (e.g., 50 to 100 mg/day). The initial response usually is very rapid, and the infection can often be clinically eradicated. However, with

TABLE 6. *Drugs Used to Treat Oral Candidiasis**

Topical
Amphotericin B oral solution
Nystatin suspension and pastilles
Clotrimazole troches
Gentian violet*
Boric acid*
Systemic
Ketoconazole (tablets)
Fluconazole (tablets and solution)
Itraconazole (capsules and solution)
Amphotericin B (intravenous)†

*Selection depends on immune status of the host, severity of the infection, and the species of *Candida* isolated.

*Renewed use of these agents has occurred, primarily in those with mucosal candidiasis resistant to other antifungal drugs.

†Usually reserved for treating recalcitrant thrush in patients with end stage AIDS and lack of response to other topical and systemically administered drugs.

subsequent relapses, higher doses of fluconazole, up to 1,200 mg/day or more, are required and partial responses at best are seen. *In vitro* susceptibility testing of the fungi recovered at these later stages shows an increase in MIC for fluconazole to more than 64 μg/ml in many of these isolates. Thus, both clinical and microbiological resistance has been observed with these yeasts.

Options for treatment of superficial candidiasis caused by fluconazole-resistant *Candida* are limited. A switch from the initial azole to a different one can be tried but is not always successful. Adding flucytosine (75 to 100 mg/kg/day in four divided doses), if clinically feasible (such as in patients with adequate bone marrow reserve), is another option. When all else fails, intravenously administered amphotericin B (approximately 0.6 mg/kg/day) has been effective in most, but not all patients. In patients with AIDS, it has always been postulated that improvement of the underlying immunological deficits might increase responsiveness to the antifungal therapy of resistant thrush. Indeed, the experience with potent antiretroviral drugs, such as the protease inhibitors, suggests that these drugs are important correlates in maintaining responsiveness to antifungal drugs in this clinical setting. Anecdotal experience also suggests that older therapies, such as gentian violet, might be of some use in patients not responding to other antifungal drugs.

In patients with dentures, good hygiene of the dental appliances is important to eradicate a potential reservoir of the organisms and subsequent relapse of infection. Chlorhexidine soaks of the dentures have been used with some success.

Candida Esophagitis

Clinical

Esophageal candidiasis may occur with oropharyngeal candidiasis, or as an isolated finding. The risk factors associated with esophagitis are the same as those for oropharyngeal candidiasis. This condition is especially frequent in patients with AIDS. Symptoms include substernal chest pain, painful swallowing and feelings of food sticking when being swallowed. Patients may complain of nausea and vomiting. The diagnosis is made by histopathologic examination and culture of tissue obtained during endoscopic examination. A suggestive appearance on barium swallow with ulcerations and an irregular mucosa may be enough to start presumptive therapy. However, since both herpes simplex virus and cytomegalovirus can produce the same clinical and radiographic picture as *Candida,* and appropriate therapy is available for all of these agents, it is important to document to the best extent possible the etiology of the patient's illness before embarking on therapy.

Diagnosis

Diagnosis of *Candida* esophagitis is made with the visualization or isolation of the fungus from biopsy specimens taken from the involved areas of the esophagus. Symptoms and x-rays are nonspecific, thus making the identification of the fungus is important to confirm the clinical impression, to select appropriate therapy, and to evaluate whether renewed symptoms after initially successful therapy are due to relapse, reinfection, or a new infection with a different organism. It is important to rule out concomitant bacterial or viral infection in patients thought to have *Candida* esophagitis.

Treatment

Candida esophagitis responds most favorably to systemic therapy; topical therapy is not as reliably effective. Patients experience symptomatic relief within several days following appropriate treatment. Fluconazole (200 to 400 mg daily) may be considered the drug of choice in most patients, but responses to ketoconazole (200 to 400 mg/day), and itraconazole (200 to 400 mg/day), are also expected. Topical therapy may be effective but mycological cure rates are lower than those obtained with the absorbable antifungal drugs. Itraconazole oral solution, a liquid formulation of itraconazole in cyclodextrin, combines the positive aspects of systemic absorption with topical action, since the solution is thick and sticks to the oral mucosa. An increasing number of patients, especially those with late-stage AIDS, may become refractory to azole therapy; intravenous amphotericin B (0.4 to 0.8 mg/kg/day) may offer some relief to these patients.

Candida Vulvovaginitis and Balanitis

Clinical

Vulvovaginal candidiasis is another mucosal infection caused by *Candida* species. While women who are diabetic, pregnant, or taking antibiotics are at increased risk for the development of this infection, often no predisposing factors can be elicited. Chronic vaginitis associated with oral candidiasis may be a presentation in HIV-infected women. Up to three quarters of women may suffer from at least one episode of vaginal candidiasis in their lifetime. A small proportion of women may suffer from repeated bouts of vaginal candidiasis, and these patients remain therapeutic challenges. The mechanisms responsible for continuously relapsing symptoms of *Candida* vaginitis are not clear, contributing to the difficulty in effectively managing this problem.

Patients may present with vaginal soreness or severe itching of the vulva. Erythema of the vagina and labia are present and may extend onto the perineum. A thick white discharge is usually evident, but some patients may have minimal discharge.

Balanitis has been associated with diabetes mellitus in males. It also may occur in the sexual partners of women with *Candida* vulvovaginitis. Symptoms include itching, erythema, and vesiculopustules on the glans penis or the foreskin.

Diagnosis

Diagnosis is dependent on observing yeast, usually in the presence of pseudohyphae and hyphae (for *C. albicans*) in the vaginal discharge. A slide prepared with one drop of 10% KOH and the discharge will be satisfactory for demonstration of the fungus. However, in order to see *Trichomonas*, which may elicit similar symptoms, a wet preparation should be made, since KOH will kill the parasite.

Treatment

Either topical agents (e.g., nystatin and clotrimazole suppositories) or oral azole therapy are effective in the treatment of vaginal candidiasis. Most recently, a one-time dose of fluconazole, 150 mg, has proved to be efficacious and well tolerated in the treatment of this condition. Consideration should be given to treating the sexual partners of women who have received treatment for *Candida* vaginitis, since the yeast may reside on the partner's penis, in either an asymptomatic or symptomatic (e.g., balanitis) state. While not currently approved for this indication in the United States, itraconazole is another alternative if the other agents cannot be used.

Primary Cutaneous Candidiasis

Clinical

These manifestations of candidiasis are superficial and should not be confused with the skin lesions secondary to hematogenous dissemination of the fungus. Superficial candidiasis may be generalized, with lesions over most of the body, but especially prominent in areas with skin folds. Alternatively, the disease can be localized to skin folds (e.g., axilla, inguinal region, and under the breasts), a condition particularly common in obese women with diabetes. *Candida* also can cause isolated and focal folliculitis and infection of the web spaces of the fingers and toes, which may be confused with infection due to dermatophytes. Diaper rash in infants may be caused by infection with *Candida*.

Diagnosis

Scrapings of lesions for KOH slide preparation and culture are recommended for the definitive diagnosis of suspicious skin lesions. The characteristic budding yeast will be visible, as may pseudohyphae and hyphae in the case of *C. albicans*.

Treatment

Topical therapy with antifungal powders, creams, or ointments should be satisfactory in most cases. In areas predisposed to moisture and skin maceration, antifungal powders, such as miconazole, are preferred. Fluconazole or itraconazole can be used if systemic therapy is required due to a lack of response to topical therapy, or if the clinical situation warrants more aggressive treatment of the skin lesions. Response to therapy usually occurs within several days and should be continued for 5 to 7 days after all signs of infection have cleared.

Onychomycosis and Paronychia

Clinical

Fungal involvement of the nail can be caused by *Candida* or dermatophytic fungi. The nail becomes discolored and disfigured with buildup of the nail. As the nailbed becomes involved, the nail may spontaneously loosen and can subsequently be lost. Onychomycosis can occur without more generalized involvement of the surrounding skin or other areas of the hands or feet.

Patients with paronychia most often present with a localized area of pain, redness, and swelling adjacent to the nailbed, but the process can extend under the nail. It is a common condition in people who frequently have their hands in water. Diabetics are also prone to this infection. A bacterial cause should be ruled out since treatment is different for the two conditions. Clinically, differentiation between bacterial etiologies and involvement with *Candida* cannot be made.

Diagnosis

Scrapings of the nail obtained with a scalpel and placed in a drop of KOH will show the characteristic yeast and pseudohyphae of *Candida* species. Scrapings should also be sent for culture to confirm the diagnosis. Aspiration of pus from a paronychia will be positive on smear and culture for *Candida*, but bacteria may also be present.

Treatment

Once distinguished from dermatophytic infection, onychomycosis is best treated with systemic therapy. Fluconazole or itraconazole have been effective, but treatment must continue for months to give time for normal nail to grow and to replace the infected and deformed nail plate. Many dosage schedules have been proposed, but fluconazole or itraconazole, 200 mg daily, is one of the more common regimens. Pulse therapy has also been used with some success. Fluconazole, 200 to 400 mg, or itraconazole, 200 mg, once weekly for 2 to 4 months may be particularly effective, but the patient must be compliant. As a general rule, onychomycosis of the fingernails is more easily treated than infection of toenails.

Treatment of paronychia involves local care, with warm soaks several times daily and antifungal therapy. Systemic therapy with fluconazole, 200 to 400 mg daily, is quite effective. Itraconazole, 200 mg daily, also may be used. Drainage of the area by means of an incision or aspiration with a needle may provide instant relief of pain and should be considered in lesions that appear amenable to this therapeutic approach.

Chronic Mucocutaneous Candidiasis

Clinical

This is a rare disease thought to be caused by a defect in the cell-mediated immune response. Patients may have repeated episodes of skin and mucous membrane involvement with *Candida,* and response to therapy may be slow. Scalp, hands, and face commonly are involved with large disfiguring lesions. Most patients present in childhood or adolescence. About 50% of patients may have associated endocrinopathies, especially Addison's disease and hypoparathyroidism. Diabetes mellitus and hypothyroidism also have been described in these patients. This disease also has been associated with abnormalities of the teeth, thymoma, chronic infection with dermatophytes, and vitiligo.

Diagnosis

Diagnosis is dependent on establishing the chronicity of severe skin and mucosal lesions that have been identified as being caused by *Candida* species (usually *C. albicans*). The presence of the associated conditions described above lends weight to the diagnosis.

Treatment

Development of disseminated candidiasis is rare. Long-term treatment with azoles results in the suppression of active candidiasis in most patients. Most published experience has been with ketoconazole, but fluconazole and itraconazole are better tolerated and presumably would be at least as efficacious in treating this disease. The role of cytokine therapy is being investigated. Relapse is common once therapy is discontinued.

INVASIVE CANDIDIASIS

Invasive candidiasis has also been called systemic candidiasis or disseminated candidiasis. However, some manifestations of this form of candidiasis appear to be localized, such as endophthalmitis, arthritis, osteomyelitis, or endocarditis. However, it is obvious that the fungus had to be transported to the site of infection, probably through the circulatory system. Thus, these otherwise focal-appearing infections can be considered manifestations of disseminated disease.

Hematogenously Disseminated Candidiasis

Clinical

This term has been suggested as the preferred nomenclature for forms of candidiasis that are spread through the bloodstream. As such, it also includes the increasingly common entity of candidemia. *Candida* species now represent the third most common organisms causing nosocomial bloodstream infections in hospitals in the United States.

In the past, candidemia was often thought of as transient or benign and thus did not require any specific management. The presence of *Candida* in the blood was thought to reflect a contaminated intravenous catheter, and once the catheter was removed, no other treatment was given. However, studies have shown that the mortality rate of patients with candidemia is much higher than in patients without positive blood cultures, thus underscoring the seriousness of candidemia. In addition, the attributable mortality (the mortality directly caused by *Candida*) is approximately 40%. Recent evidence suggests, moreover, that candidemia is neither a sensitive nor specific indicator of serious candidal infection. For example, approximately 50% of patients with organ-invasive candidiasis will have negative blood cultures. On the other hand, not all patients with candidemia will have evidence of deep-seated infection. It is impossible to identify which patients are truly infected and who had positive blood cultures following colonization of the intravenous catheter and subsequent seeding of other organs using the most recent techniques. Thus, all patients with *Candida* in their blood need to be fully evaluated and managed aggressively to avoid both acute effects of the infection and long-term sequelae.

Diagnosis

The major problem in the definitive diagnosis of invasive candidiasis is distinguishing between colonization and actual infection. As the population of patients at risk becomes more immunosuppressed and instrumented with greater frequency, the distinctions blur, since many patients colonized with *Candida* species will develop invasive disease due to their critically ill state. Thus, treatment is warranted before full-blown actual tissue invasion occurs to decrease the morbidity and mortality associated with unmistakable clinical infection. Strategies to evaluate this approach are being studied.

Blood cultures are neither very sensitive nor specific as indicators of invasive candidiasis. Approximately 50% of patients with organ-invasive candidiasis never have positive blood cultures. In contrast, an undetermined number of patients with positive blood cultures, especially when these are clearly related to intravenous catheter infection, will have no serious sequelae from the presence of *Candida* in their blood. However, it has become increasingly clear over the past several years that it is impossible to accurately predict who will not need therapy because of (1) the acute or long-term effects of the candidemia and (2) whether it was a truly transient and benign event. The concept of "transient" candidemia was developed at a time when patients were less critically ill than patients treated in the 1990s. Hence, the more striking acuity of illness, combined with procedures and advanced supportive measures, enhance susceptibility to the development of invasive candidiasis. At present, there is no way to identify thosc patients in whom candidemia truly is transient and thus representative of a benign condition.

Should clinical evidence for involvement of specific regions of the body become apparent (i.e., back pain indicative of vertebral osteomyelitis or eye pain and decreased visual acuity indicative of endophthalmitis) appropriate studies should be done. In the case of viscera and bones, CT and MRI scans have been very useful and may indicate the presence of one or more space-occupying lesions.

Involvement of the eye is manifested by white lesions on the retina that progress anteriorly, resulting in clouding of the vitreous. Vitrectomy is often required for diagnostic and therapeutic purposes. Yeasts can be seen on smears of the vitreous, and the organism may grow from the biopsy specimen.

Treatment

Amphotericin B, 0.5 to 1 mg/kg/day, has been the mainstay of treatment for all forms of invasive candidiasis. However, randomized trials of fluconazole in doses of at least 400 mg daily, have shown fluconazole to be comparable to amphotericin B in treating candidemia. Thus, in most patients it is reasonable to begin treating with fluconazole. If *C. krusei* is recovered from the blood, a switch to amphotericin B is warranted. On the other hand, if another *Candida* species is found to have an elevated MIC *in vitro* and the patient is doing well, it is unclear whether a change in therapy is warranted. Studies evaluating higher doses of fluconazole (e.g., 800 mg/day), with and without amphotericin B, are in progress, and may provide a therapeutic approach that will improve the prognosis of this serious disease. Itraconazole has yet to be studied for the treatment of this form of candidiasis.

Hepatosplenic candidiasis

Clinical

This is a distinct clinical syndrome occurring in patients who have recovered from chemotherapy-induced neutropenia. Patients may have had an episode of candidemia during the period of neutropenia, and they may have been treated with amphotericin B during this time. As the neutrophil count increases, the patient continues to exhibit fever, often hectic in pattern, anorexia, and right upper quadrant abdominal pain.

Diagnosis

The white blood cell count increases to above normal values, and the liver function tests become abnormal. While transaminases are increased several-fold over top normal values, disproportionate increases in alkaline phosphatase and bilirubin are often seen. Scanning of the abdomen shows round lesions in liver and often in the spleen and kidney. These may enhance when imaged with contrast agents. Typical "target lesions" are often seen on ultrasound or CT scanning of the liver.

Biopsy of the lesion may be needed to make the diagnosis, since other infectious causes and leukemic infiltration can cause similar lesions. However, the characteristic clinical syndrome when all of the above features are present makes the diagnosis of hepatosplenic candidiasis much more likely. Biopsy shows neutrophilic infiltrate and very few organisms. Thus, hepatosplenic candidiasis may be present, even though Gram stain and other stains and culture may be negative. However, it can be useful to have ruled out other causes for the clinical syndrome.

Treatment

Hepatosplenic candidiasis is often quite refractory to treatment with amphotericin B. In contrast, fluconazole, 400 to 800 mg daily, has been quite effective in controlling this infection. Patients typically defervesce and regain a feeling of well-being within 14 days after fluconazole therapy is begun. The role of itraconazole for this indication is not known.

Suppurative Thrombophlebitis

Clinical

This infection usually occurs in the setting of a patient with an intravenous catheter that has become infected with *Candida* species. A disproportionate number of *C. parapsilosis* are recovered from these infections. The catheter may be in a central vein, and the major veins of the chest may become clotted with infected material. The clinical presentation depends on the area affected. If a peripheral vein in an arm is infected, the patient may develop swelling and pain in that extremity. A red, tender cord, reflecting the distended vein with internal thrombus may be palpable. Involvement of central veins, such as internal jugular or subclavian veins, will present with similar local symptoms; signs and swelling of the head and neck can occur if venous return from those areas is impeded. Patients will usually be febrile and may appear septic if the infection is rapidly progressive. In this instance, blood cultures are usually positive.

Diagnosis

The characteristic sequence of events described above is highly suggestive of the diagnosis. Most often the differential diagnostic problem is determining if the clinically obvious clot is infected. Blood cultures are important to obtain; two a day for 2 or 3 days are often sufficient. If possible, the intravenous catheter should be removed and the tip of the catheter then cultured. This will often grow the offending microorganism and support the clinical impression that the clot is infected.

Treatment

Amphotericin B, 0.6 to 1 mg/kg/day, or fluconazole, 400 to 800 mg/day, should be used as initial therapy pending identification of the causative organism. Given that these patients are usually quite ill, intravenous therapy is preferred if fluconazole is the drug of choice; a change to oral administration can be made when the patient has improved. Catheter removal is important and will result in clinical improvement in and of itself. Surgical debridement of the infected vein with removal of the clot is also beneficial when it can be safely performed. Otherwise, modification of antifungal therapy is similar to that outlined for the treatment of candidemia.

Endophthalmitis

Clinical

Patients with *Candida* endophthalmitis present with eye pain, blurred vision, or loss of sight. While the infection undoubtedly results as a consequence of candidemia, only about 50% of patients will have a prior history of candidemia. Endophthalmitis can occur concomitant with positive blood cultures as a manifestation of the acute infection, or it may occur as a late sequela within several months of the episode of candidemia. The lesions begin as a chorioretinitis, and the effects on vision will depend on the location of the lesion with respect to the macula.

Diagnosis

Lesions caused by *Candida* appear on the retina as cottony white patches, which grow anteriorly into the vitreous as the lesion progresses. Once vitreal involvement is demonstrated, manifested as clouding of the posterior chamber, a decision needs to be made whether vitreal biopsy should be done. Gram stain and culture of the vitreous may provide evidence for the presence of the yeasts, but may be negative even in definitive cases. The presence of a positive blood culture is supporting evidence for the etiology of the infection.

Treatment

Infections due to *C. albicans* can be treated with fluconazole, 400 to 800 mg/day, although clinical experience with this agent has been limited. Addition of flucytosine, 100 to 150 mg/kg/day, may increase the efficacy of fluconazole. More experience has accrued with amphotericin B, with or without flucytosine, but results have been variable. While the role of vitrectomy is controversial, it may be useful for making a diagnosis in cases without clear etiology. A multidisciplinary approach, including input from specialists in eye diseases and infectious diseases is important to provide the most-up-to-date therapy for this devastating condition.

Osteomyelitis

Clinical

Candidal infection of bone can be secondary to hematogenous dissemination or direct inoculation, such as following trauma, or less commonly, surgery. Virtually any bone can be involved, but vertebrae are most commonly affected following an episode of candidemia. When the spine is involved, intervertebral discs also commonly are infected. Manifestations are nonspecific and include pain and swelling of the involved area. Fever, night sweats, and anorexia may also occur.

Diagnosis

At the time of diagnosis of the bone infection, blood cultures are usually negative. Biopsy of the involved bone is required to make a definitive diagnosis, and cultures usually are positive if adequate tissue is sent to the laboratory.

Treatment

Fluconazole has been successful in treating candidal osteomyelitis. Doses of 400 to 800 mg/day are used most commonly. Treatment duration is uncertain, but many experts would continue therapy for at least 6 to 12 months beyond resolution of clinical symptoms and signs of infection. Infections caused by fluconazole-resistant *Candida* may be treated with amphotericin B, although long-term administration of intravenous therapy is problematic. The role of itraconazole is not clear, but should be effective in many cases. Antifungal susceptibility testing may help in deciding which drug to use, but interpretation of results should be made in conjunction with an expert in the performance and interpretation of these tests.

Arthritis

Clinical

Joint involvement is secondary to hematogenous dissemination, contiguous spread from infected bone, or direct implantation following trauma. Patients with *Candida* infection of the joints develop effusion, pain, swelling, and warmth around the involved joint. Large joints, such as knees and shoulders, are commonly involved. Nonspecific symptoms, such as fever, night sweats, and anorexia, may also be present.

Diagnosis

This is most easily accomplished following recovery of the organism from synovial fluid. Occasionally, synovial biopsy may be necessary, and Gram stain will show the presence of an acute inflammatory response along with the budding yeasts. Blood cultures may be helpful in determining if the septic arthritis is part of a more disseminated infection.

Treatment

The same principles apply to the treatment of candidal arthritis as pertain to the treatment of osteomyelitis and other disseminated forms of candidiasis. Fluconazole, 400 to 800 mg/day, is useful for chronic therapy, which may last for 6 to 12 months, depending on any underlying illnesses and the response of the patient to therapy. Intravenous amphotericin B also is useful, but its long-term use is problematic. There is little reason to use intra-articular injections of amphotericin B, especially since amphotericin B is quite toxic to the joint space.

Peritonitis

Clinical

Candida peritonitis most often occurs in patients with perforated bowel or as a complication of continuous ambulatory peritoneal dialysis (CAPD). A ruptured abdominal viscus is often accompanied by polymicrobial soiling of the peritoneum. *Candida* spp. are frequently recovered as part of this flora. Patients may present postsurgery for bowel disease or with acute trauma to the abdomen resulting in bowel perforation. In either case, signs of peritoneal irritation predominate. Early in the infection, fever and abdominal pain may be the only indication that an infection is brewing. As the infection becomes more widespread, the characteristic signs of peritonitis, such as abdominal pain and rigidity develop. Areas of involvement may organize with the formation of abscesses.

Candida spp. are now a common cause of peritonitis in patients treated with CAPD and are especially frequent in patients who have received antibiotics for the treatment of one or more prior episodes of bacterial peritonitis. The *Candida* presumably originate from the patient's own gastrointestinal or skin flora. Fever, abdominal pain, and anorexia are common complaints. Some patients may present with low-grade fever and cloudy dialysate, but with no clinical findings of peritonitis. In these patients, infection is just beginning. The process, however, can be subacute, and many patients have nonspecific complaints of low-grade fever, anorexia, and malaise with no firm evidence for the presence of an infection. In these patients, the infection can be present for days to weeks before a diagnosis is made. Careful examination of the peritoneal dialysate for the presence of inflammatory cells and microorganisms is important in defining the etiology of the patient's complaints.

Diagnosis

In patients with ruptured bowel, culture of pus obtained at surgery is the best way to confirm the diagnosis of an infection. The yeasts are frequently seen on Gram stain and may be one of many organisms seen and recovered from cultures. In the patient with CAPD peritonitis, the peritoneal dialysate is cloudy, containing several hundred to several thousand white blood cells, predominately neutrophils. Gram stain is positive for yeast in the majority of patients and culture will be positive. If the catheter is removed and cultured, it is often culture positive as well.

Treatment

The decision to treat polymicrobial peritonitis containing bacteria and yeasts is controversial, but the clinical situation may help in making that decision. For example, a healthy young man with a gunshot wound to the abdomen may not require antifungal therapy if surgery is uncomplicated and carried out soon after the trauma. In contrast, the same microbiology seen in an elderly patient with underlying diseases and a more prolonged and complicated hospital course may indicate that the patient is at increased risk of problems associated with the isolation of *Candida* from the abdomen, including candidemia. The decision to begin antifungal treatment in this instance is more compelling. Fluconazole, 400 mg/day, should be sufficient for most patients with peritoneal candidiasis. Amphotericin B, 0.5 to 1.0 mg/kg/day given intravenously, also has been used, but is more toxic. The roles for lipid formulations of amphotericin B and itraconazole have not been established in this setting.

Patients with *Candida* peritonitis secondary to CAPD do well with fluconazole, 200 to 400 mg/day. This includes most species of *Candida,* including *C. glabrata.* Clinical experience has shown that removal of the dialysis catheter almost always is required, since leaving the catheter in place delays the clinical response and, in most cases, prevents cure of the infection with medical therapy alone. The possibility of starting therapy with fluconazole and then removing the catheter and reimplanting a new one several days later, obviating the need for interim hemodialysis, is currently under investigation. Intraperitoneal amphotericin B has been used in the past, but is toxic and usually results in the formation of adhesions, limiting the reinstitution of CAPD. Successful therapy of patients receiving CAPD should be based not only on the eradication of the infection, but on the ability of the patient to resume peritoneal dialysis without requiring hemodialysis.

Urinary Tract Candidiasis

Clinical

Candida spp. can infect the entire urinary tract. Both bladder and kidney involvement have become common problems in the care of patients. Patients with diabetes mellitus are at increased risk for developing lower urinary tract candidiasis, as well as involvement of kidney with the formation of fungus balls in the renal collecting system. In addition, other risk factors include prior antibacterial therapy, oral contraceptives, Foley catheters, and other foreign bodies in the urinary tract. Cystitis is accompanied by frequency, urgency, and dysuria, and as with urinary tract infections, in general, is more common in women. Asymptomatic candiduria is common and is often a fortuitous finding in hospitalized patients.

Upper tract involvement, pyelonephritis, presents with fever, flank pain, and symptoms of urinary tract irritation. Patients develop this manifestation of candidiasis either from hematogenous spread or following ascending infection in patients with *Candida* cystitis. When the collecting system is involved, fungus balls can occur and may lead to symptoms and signs of urinary tract obstruction.

Diagnosis

The mere presence of *Candida* in the urine does not imply active infection and may reflect colonization of the bladder, especially in patients with indwelling urinary tract catheters. However, when accompanied by clinical symptoms and white cells in the urine, the presence of yeast in the urine probably indicates active infection. The presence of white cell casts may reflect upper tract involvement. Patients may also have evidence of systemic infection, such as leukocytosis, and elevation of BUN/creatinine.

Cystitis is characterized by superficial involvement of the bladder mucosa, much the same as the findings in oropharyngeal candidiasis (thrush), and this is easily recognized on cystoscopy. Laboratory examination of urine, however, does not discriminate between active infection of upper or lower urinary tract or between simple colonization and active infection. To complicate the interpretation of culture results, there is no consensus on the number of yeasts required in the urine to define infection. Thus, greater than 10^3, 10^4, or 10^5 yeasts/ml of urine is of no diagnostic significance.

Treatment

In patients with asymptomatic candiduria, at least two cultures should be obtained on different days before deciding whether therapy is indicated. If the patient has an indwelling bladder catheter, this should be removed and not replaced if possible. If the patient is asymptomatic, no further treatment may be needed. If the candiduria does not spontaneously resolve, some controversy exists as to the best way to proceed. Fluconazole, 200 to 400 mg/day for 5 to 14 days has been suggested as an effective but relatively nontoxic approach to medical therapy. Similarly, amphotericin B bladder irrigation, 50 mg in 500 to 1,000 ml 5% dextrose in water for 3 to 10 days, has also been advocated for use. However, the manipulation of the bladder catheter enhances the risk for superinfection. With either method, relapse or recurrent candiduria occurs in at least 50% of patients, so the long-term value of treating asymptomatic candiduria is not clear. Reversal of predisposing factors is probably the most efficacious way to eradicate the positive cultures.

In patients with symptomatic candiduria, it is often difficult to determine whether the infection represents bladder or kidney involvement. In either case, fluconazole, 200 to 400 mg/day, has proven useful in controlling and curing the infection. Foreign bodies should be removed from the urinary tract, if possible. Treatment for approximately 1 week following resolution of signs of infection should suffice. Urine culture should be obtained at the end of therapy and 1 month later, if clinically indicated.

Fungus balls in the urinary tract should be removed either endoscopically or during an open surgical procedure. Medical therapy alone is unsuccessful in almost all patients, but suppressive therapy with fluconazole is often used in those patients who cannot tolerate a surgical procedure.

Endocarditis

Clinical

Candida spp. are the most common fungal causes of endocarditis. The infection is rare, but increasing in incidence given the increase in the number of patients with prosthetic heart valves. While native valve involvement does occur, the infection is much more common on prostheses. Most of the cases occur following cardiac surgery for valve replacement, but intravenous drug abusers are also susceptible to infecting their heart valves with this fungus.

The presenting signs and symptoms of candidal endocarditis are nonspecific and include fever, malaise, shortness of breath, and palpitations. New cardiac murmurs are important clues to the diagnosis. Congestive heart failure and systemic emboli are complications that can occur at any time during the course of the infection.

Diagnosis

Blood cultures from patients with *Candida* endocarditis are almost always positive, and if emboli are removed from peripheral vessels, culture of the clot is usually positive as well. Echocardiography can demonstrate large vegetations on the valves and valve perforations and cardiac abscesses can also be observed.

Treatment

Valve replacement is the most important therapeutic intervention in the vast majority of patients with *Candida* endocarditis. Fluconazole, 400 to 800 mg/day, may be used as initial therapy, but many would start with amphotericin B, approximately 0.8 mg/kg/day, and switch to fluconazole after the acute infection is controlled. The addition of flucytosine to either of these regimens is of unproven value but is often done. In patients with infection of native valves, therapy for 6 to 12 months should be curative; however, in patients with prosthetic valvular infection, lifelong suppressive therapy with fluconazole is reasonable.

Myocardium

Clinical

Involvement of the heart muscle by *Candida* spp. is usually part of a more disseminated infection. Pericardium may also be involved in the course of the infection. Symptoms of heart failure can develop, but the only manifestation of myocardial involvement may be nonspecific changes of the electrocardiogram. A variety of dysrhythmias can occur, depending on the location of the cardiac lesions.

Diagnosis

Echocardiograms may show lesions compatible with abscesses and, when present in patients with disseminated candidiasis or candidemia, should raise the suspicion that the lesions are secondary to candidal infection. Definitive diagnosis is dependent upon isolation of the fungus from the lesions. For practical purposes, however, cardiac involvement in the setting of active candidal infection is usually enough for a presumptive diagnosis.

Treatment

The same principles for the medical therapy of disseminated candidiasis and candidemia apply (see page 46). Surgical drainage of abscesses may be required, but the decision for surgical intervention needs to be individualized according to the entire clinical picture.

Central Nervous System

Meningitis

Clinical

Meningeal involvement can be part of disseminated candidiasis or as an isolated clinical finding. *Candida* spp. may infect cerebrospinal fluid shunts or follow neurosurgical procedures. Typical symptoms and signs of meningitis occur: headache, nausea, vomiting, photophobia. Meningismus and signs of meningeal irritation may also occur.

Diagnosis

CSF pleocytosis is the rule in patients with candidal meningitis. Cells can be predominantly lymphocytes or neutrophils: 50% of patients will present with either cell type predominating. CSF glucose is usually decreased and protein is increased. Yeasts may be seen on Gram stain of CSF and culture, which is the only method to definitively diagnose the infection. In India ink preparations of the CSF, *Candida* will appear as nonencapsulated budding yeasts.

Treatment

Most experience has been with amphotericin B, approximately 1 mg/kg/day, usually with flucytosine, 100 to 150 mg/kg/day. However, fluconazole or amphotericin B plus fluconazole can be considered for initial therapy in patients with active acute infection. Intrathecal administration of antifungal drugs, especially amphotericin B, is thought to be unnecessary and should be reserved for special circumstances, such as the patient with an intraventricular shunt that cannot be removed. However, it is clear that the removal of foreign bodies, such as shunts, maximizes both the rate of response to treatment, as well as the ultimate end result of control of the infection. Insufficient experience with the use of liposomal preparations of amphotericin B limits their recommendation as initial agents. However, since good responses have been seen in patients with cryptococcal meningitis, by extrapolation, these formulations should also be effective in treating candidal meningitis. The most appropriate duration of therapy is unknown, but treatment usually will extend for 1 year or longer.

Brain Abscess

Clinical

Both microabscesses and larger abscesses have been reported to occur secondary to parenchymal brain infection with *Candida* spp., usually as part of disseminated infection. Symptoms and signs are dependent on the location of such lesions, but virtually any neurological syndrome can occur following brain infection with this fungus.

Diagnosis

Lesions may appear as typical abscesses on CT or MRI scans. CSF may be abnormal, with evidence of parameningeal focus (sterile cultures, but with CSF pleocytosis, elevated protein, and decreased glucose) or evidence of meningitis (positive CSF cultures).

Treatment

Principles for therapy are the same as for disseminated candidiasis, candidemia, and *Candida* meningitis. The relative role of amphotericin B versus fluconazole is unclear, but fluconazole, in doses in excess of 400 mg/day should be effective in the treatment of infections caused by susceptible organisms. Treatment duration will usually be 6 to 12 months, but the exact duration of therapy to achieve cure is unknown.

Pneumonia

Clinical

Candidal pneumonia is rare and is usually a manifestation of disseminated candidiasis. Fever and sputum positive for *Candida* are not diagnostic for *Candida* pneumonia, since the yeasts may simply reflect colonization of the oropharynx with the organism. Patients with disseminated candidiasis and lung involvement usually have multiple diffuse small nodular lesions in a miliary pattern. Respiratory symptoms, such as dyspnea and cough, are found, as well as fever. It is distinctly unusual to implicate aspiration as a cause of *Candida* pneumonia and in the proper setting, the much more common bacterial causes of aspiration pneumonia should be sought.

Diagnosis

Given the problems in interpreting cultures that are potentially contaminated with oropharyngeal secretions, sputum and specimens obtained through a bronchoscope are unreliable. Thus, only open lung biopsy or percutaneous aspiration of pulmonary lesions provide suitable material for a definitive diagnosis. In patients with disseminated candidiasis, however, a presumptive diagnosis of *Candida* pneumonia can be made if respiratory status declines in concert with the development of other manifestations of candidal infection in the acutely ill patient. Blood cultures are therefore useful in supporting the clinical impression.

Treatment

Amphotericin B, 0.6 to 1.0 mg/kg/day, or fluconazole, 400 to 800 mg/day, for use in treating disseminated candidiasis should also suffice in treating candidal pneumonia. Duration of therapy will usually be on the order of weeks, and should continue for at least 5 to 10 days beyond the last evidence of active infection.

5

Cryptococcus

Clinical

Once considered a rare disease seen in patients such as those receiving corticosteroids, cryptococcosis is now occurring with much greater frequency. It occurs in patients with AIDS as well as those with other causes of suppression of their cell-mediated immunity, such as patients with lymphoma, T-cell leukemia, chronic lymphocytic leukemia, and graft-versus-host disease. In industrial countries, up to 10% of patients with AIDS may develop this disease and in developing countries, such as in Africa, the disease is found in up to one-half of HIV-infected patients. Unlike most other opportunistic fungal infections, cryptococcosis is rarely associated with neutropenia. Like many fungal pathogens, cryptococcosis is initially a pulmonary pathogen, inhaled into the lungs from environmental sources. The association of pigeons and cryptococcosis is well appreciated, but it is the ability of pigeon droppings to fertilize the soil that encourages the growth of *Cryptococcus neoformans*. The birds themselves do not become ill.

Cryptococcus neoformans exists as two varieties, *C. neoformans* var. *neoformans* and *C. neoformans* var. *gatti*. Important differences are found in the virulence and epidemiology of these isolates. *C. neoformans* var. *neoformans* is the variety responsible for the vast majority of infections and may be isolated from soil in most areas of the world. It is a true opportunistic pathogen unlike *C. neoformans* var. *gatti*, which appears to be a primary pathogen, much like *Coccidioides immitis* or *Histoplasma capsulatum*. *C. neoformans* var. *gatti* grows selectively under particular species of eucalyptus trees and thus is found only in certain tropical areas of the world, such as southern California, parts of Africa, and Australia. In addition to immunocompromised patients, cryptococcosis caused by variety *gatti* occurs in nonimmunocompromised patients and may be more refractory to treatment than disease caused by variety *neoformans*. Thus, cryptococci should be identified by the laboratory as completely as possible.

Cryptococcosis may present as a chronic, subacute to acute pulmonary, meningeal, or systemic disease. Patients with pulmonary cryptococcosis are often asymptomatic, but when the disease is present, symptoms include pleuritic chest pain, cough, and low-grade fever. Patients with chronic pulmonary disease are at increased risk for dissemination to the central nervous system. Up to 85% of cases of cryptococcal infection involve the brain and meninges. Symptoms usually develop slowly over time, and may include headache, dizziness, irritability, confusion, nausea, and vomiting, as well as focal neurological deficits. Acute onset can occur in the severely immunocompromised patient. Cutaneous infection, secondary to dissemination, occurs in up to 15% of patients, and usually is associated with a poor prognosis.

On occasion, a focus of cryptococcal involvement, referred to as a cryptococcoma, can present as a solitary mass. These lesions may occur in any organ, but most frequently in the lungs or brain. They can be confused with other infectious processes or malignancy. In order to make a definitive diagnosis, a biopsy usually is needed.

Diagnosis

Cryptococcosis is one the easiest mycoses to diagnose. Using India ink, CSF and other body fluids should be examined microscopically for the presence of encapsulated budding yeast cells (Fig. 3). However, some strains of *C. neoformans* from HIV-infected patients may appear to be only slightly encapsulated or capsule-deficient. Culture of the fungus from any source is indicative of cryptococcal infection. The use of cryptococcal antigen testing of serum and CSF is extremely useful since the test is sensitive and specific, and now the method of choice for diagnosing cryptococcal meningitis. In HIV-positive patients, the CSF antigen titers tend to exceed those seen in other infected populations, and dilutions into the millions are common.

Treatment

Prognosis of patients with cryptococcal meningitis is highly dependent on mental status, acuity of disease on presentation, and underlying diseases. Patients with AIDS and organ transplant recipients, by virtue of their irreversible immunosuppression, are rarely, if ever, cured. In

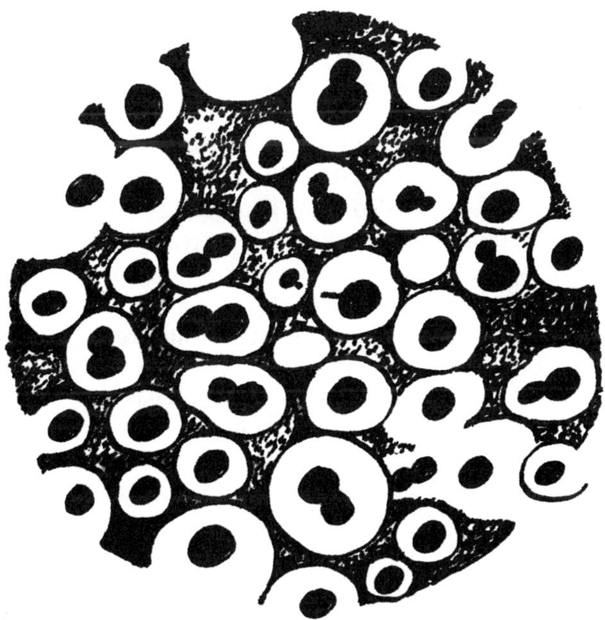

FIG. 3. Appearance of *Cryptococcus neoformans* in an India ink preparation.

contrast, patients without continuous immunosuppression can be cured and this should be the goal of therapy for them. In the pre-AIDS era, several studies evaluated the combination of amphotericin B and flucytosine for treating cryptococcal meningitis; several different regimens of treatment have been evaluated in the AIDS patient. Since the results of therapy in renal transplant patients were so poor with amphotericin B plus flucytosine, many physicians treat these organ transplant patients in a manner similar to those with AIDS, with long-term, if not life-long, suppressive therapy.

AIDS and Organ Transplant Patients

If the patient is merely complaining of headache and has a normal mental status, treatment with an oral regimen of fluconazole, 400 to 800 mg/day can be tried. However, most authorities would now start therapy with amphotericin B, 0.7 mg/kg/day, for at least 2 weeks and then switch to therapy with fluconazole, 400 mg/day. Adding flucytosine in the first 2 weeks of therapy does not appear to enhance the effectiveness of the regimen. However, the relapse rate in patients who have received 2 weeks of flucytosine appears to be less than that seen in patients treated without flucytosine.

In the patient completely intolerant of amphotericin B, an entirely oral regimen of fluconazole (400 to 800 mg/day plus flucytosine, 100 to 150 mg/kg/day in four divided doses) can be used, and has resulted in an impressive response rate of over 80%. Patients with lethargy or other mental status changes will need to be treated with amphotericin B until their condition has stabilized.

It is still too early to determine the role of liposomal amphotericin B in AIDS and organ transplant patients with cryptococcal disease and such use should be restricted to clinical investigation until more information is available.

Non-AIDS Patients

Combination therapy with amphotericin B (0.4 mg/kg/day plus flucytosine, 150 mg/kg/day in four divided doses) has been the traditionally used therapy. However, experience has shown that this regimen results in failure in at least 25% of patients so treated. The dose of amphotericin B has been considered too low and the dose of flucytosine too high. Therefore, a combined regimen of amphotericin B (0.5 to 0.8 mg/kg/day) and flucytosine (75 to 100 mg/kg/day in four divided doses) may be preferred but no firm information is available to support this recommendation. Similarly, the role of oral azoles in the therapy of these patients is unclear. While there is no doubt that fluconazole and itraconazole would be effective treatment of cryptococcal meningitis in the non-AIDS patients, the optimal duration of therapy is unknown and may be longer than that of the previously mentioned regimens of amphotericin B and flucytosine. If azole therapy is to be used, it would seem prudent to continue therapy for at least 4 weeks beyond all resolution of symptoms, CSF and blood culture negativity, and low, stable levels of cryptococcal antigen titers (but preferably negative). Because of drug interactions and specific requirements for optimal absorption of itraconazole, fluconazole is the preferred azole for initial use in this setting. The average patient so treated will require a minimum of 6 to 10 weeks of therapy.

In the non-AIDS population, as with the AIDS patient, the role of liposomal amphotericin B preparations in treating cryptococcal disease is unclear and should be considered investigational for now.

6

Pseudallescheria (Scedosporium)

Clinical

Pseudallescheria boydii has been known by a variety of names (*Petriellidium boydii* and *Allescheria boydii*), complicating its recognition as an important fungal pathogen. Two points are significant about this fungus. It is the only pathogenic fungus primarily virulent in its telomorph (sexual) form and it is inherently resistant to amphotericin B. Recently, it has been recognized that the anamorph (asexual) form, *Scedosporium apiospermum,* is also a cause of infection. This fungus was once known as *Monosporium apiospermum.* A closely related organism, *Scedosporium prolificans* (*inflatum*) has also been implicated as a cause of human infection.

Infection with *Pseudallescheria* occurs in immunocompetent and immunocompromised hosts. In normal hosts, mycetoma is the usual presentation of the disease following a penetrating injury. Lesions can appear on skin, in bone, brain, or joints, depending on the location of the traumatic event. Lesions are subacute in duration and incite a pyogenic inflammatory response. Infection of a preexisting cavity has also been noted. Cases of pulmonary pseudallescheriosis and central nervous system infections have been reported in victims of near-drowning episodes. Finally, this fungus can produce a spectrum of illnesses similar to *Aspergillus,* such as invasive sinusitis, external otitis, bronchial hypersensitivity mimicking bronchopulmonary aspergillosis, invasive pulmonary disease, and disseminated infection.

Prolonged neutropenia and corticosteroid therapy are the major predispositions to the development of pseudallescheriosis. In these patients, the disease often begins in the lungs and may disseminate from there. Clinically, it is indistinguishable from infection caused by *Aspergillus* spp. or *Fusarium* spp.

Diagnosis

Diagnosis of pseudallescheriosis is based on culture of the fungus from biopsy specimens. Histologically, the organism is indistinguishable from *Aspergillus* spp. or *Fusarium* spp., all having angular, dichotomously branching, septate hyphae in tissue (Fig. 1). Given the need for different therapies for the latter two infections, it is critical to make a definitive identification of the fungus.

Treatment

Invasive infections due to *P. boydii* often carry a high mortality. The poor prognosis associated with this illness is due, at least in part, to its being highly refractory to antifungal chemotherapy, including amphotericin B. Antifungal azoles usually are recommended as the drug of choice for pseudallescheriosis, yet immunocompromised patients often fail to respond to single-agent azole therapy. Miconazole had been regarded as the first-line agent in patients with rapidly progressive life-threatening infection. However, given the toxicity and inconvenience of four daily intravenous doses of the drug, oral alternatives have been tried. As a result, most authorities would now recommend a trial of itraconazole, 200 mg bid, in patients who are not moribund. Serum concentrations should be followed to insure absorption. As measured by bioassay, concentrations of over 2 µg/ml should be sufficient, but no information is available to address this point. Alternatives to itraconazole include ketoconazole and fluconazole. Itraconazole seems to be a safer alternative than ketoconazole; there is less information about the efficacy of fluconazole in the treatment of this infection. Another recently proposed therapeutic option is combination therapy with amphotericin B plus an antifungal azole. In *in vitro* studies, augmentation of antifungal activity has been observed, but correlation with appropriate animal models or patients is currently unavailable. Duration of antifungal therapy is hard to predict, but normally would be on the order of months to years. Patients with abnormal lung anatomy may have to receive suppressive therapy for life in order to minimize disease activity, since sterilization of the lungs may be impossible. As a general rule, continuation of therapy for 3 to 6 months following resolution of clinical signs and symptoms of the infection or negative cultures from the involved area(s) seems to be a reasonable approach to the unanswered question of duration of therapy. If an isolated cutaneous mycetoma is present, surgical excision may be curative.

Infections caused by *Scedosporium* spp. also are very difficult to treat, due in part to the immunosuppressed status of patients, and also to the fact that these organisms are highly resistant to currently available antifungal agents. Most infections are treated with amphotericin B, but itraconazole or miconazole can also be tried. Consultation with experts in this area is highly recommended.

7

Fusarium

Clinical

Fusarium species are found ubiquitously and are often responsible for the decay of vegetables. In humans, these fungi were once considered to cause only localized infections of the skin, nails, and cornea. They are now recognized as a causative agent in disseminated fungal infections in immunocompromised hosts, especially those with hematologic malignancies undergoing bone marrow transplantation or intensive cytotoxic chemotherapy. The prognosis in patients with fusarial infections is often poor, related primarily to the degree of immunosuppression. Achieving cure with antifungal therapy has been very difficult and is usually impossible without a complete recovery of bone marrow function and replenishment of circulating neutrophils.

Clinical presentation of patients with fusarial infection is nonspecific. Patients will usually have prolonged neutropenia and will have persistent fever, unresponsive to antimicrobial agents. Over half will develop skin lesions that contain the fungus. This is in contrast to aspergillosis, where skin lesions are distinctly rare. If pneumonia is present, respiratory symptoms, such as dyspnea, cough, and chest pain may occur.

Diagnosis

Patients with disseminated fusarial infections often present with similar clinical characteristics as patients with disseminated aspergillosis. However, there is a higher incidence of skin and subcutaneous lesions (>60%) seen in patients with fusariosis as compared with aspergillosis. Additionally, *Fusarium* spp., unlike *Aspergillus* spp., are often recoverable from blood culture detection systems, such as lysis centrifugation. Histopathologically, the dichotomously branching, septate hyphae seen in tissue biopsy are difficult to distinguish from those seen with *Aspergillus* spp. as well as other hyalohyphomycoses, making positive cultures a necessity for establishing the diagnosis of fusariosis.

Treatment

Due to the severe immunocompromise of most patients with disseminated fusarial infections, prognosis has been poor. Amphotericin B, 1 to 1.5 mg/kg/day, has been recommended as initial therapy, but high doses of fluconazole, 800 to 1,200 mg/day, have also been used. Perhaps combinations of amphotericin B and fluconazole should be used in desperately ill patients, but there is scant evidence to support this approach. The role of liposomal formulations of amphotericin B is unknown, but since larger amounts of amphotericin B can be administered with these formulations, serious consideration should be given to their use in patients with life-threatening fusarial infections. It is critical that the bone marrow recover. With the reappearance of circulating neutrophils, the prognosis improves substantially. Thus, cytokines that facilitate bone marrow reconstitution, such as G-CSF and GM-CSF, may be tried in patients with this infection, unless there is a contraindication.

8

Agents Causing Mucormycosis

Clinical

Many species of the Mucorales cause the disease called mucormycosis. These infections are among the most aggressive and tissue destructive found in modern medicine. Rapid diagnosis is essential if the patient is to be saved and organ function is to be preserved. The most commonly recovered organism from patients with mucormycosis is *Rhizopus,* the common bread mold. *Mucor,* itself, is only responsible for a minority of cases. It is beyond the scope of this book to delve into the arcane subject of nomenclature of the different fungi causing this disease and into the naming of the disease itself, but this information can be found by the curious elsewhere (see references at the end of this book).

The most important association to remember concerning mucormycosis is that of rhinocerebral mucormycosis and diabetes mellitus. This manifestation of mucormycosis can begin with headache, low-grade fever, and signs and symptoms of sinusitis. Since most of these patients are seen by primary care health providers, these individuals should clearly recognize the potentially fatal disease incubating in diabetic patients with this presentation. If treatment for bacterial sinusitis is the therapy chosen, failure of the disease to respond within several days indicates the urgent need for aggressive diagnostic studies to search for possible fungal etiologies. Other less common predisposing factors associated with the development of mucormycosis include neutropenia, corticosteroid therapy, bone marrow or solid organ transplantation, burns, and deferoxamine therapy for the management of iron and aluminum overload (Table 7).

As the disease progresses, mucormycosis may cause blurred vision, pain behind the eye, and conjunctivitis. Later manifestations include proptosis, chemosis, extension into the hard palate with the development of a black eschar, or evidence of extension into the brain, such as

TABLE 7. *Mucormycosis Syndromes*

Manifestation	Clinical Setting
Rhinocerebral	Diabetes mellitus ± ketoacidosis; neutropenia
Central nervous system	Head trauma, severely immunocompromised patients
Pulmonary	Neutropenia secondary to cytotoxic chemotherapy
Gastrointestinal	Protein calorie malnutrition
Cutaneous	Direct trauma; contaminated wound dressings
Miscellaneous (osteomyelitis)	Dissemination from another focus, trauma

somnolence, neurologic signs, or seizures. Mucormycosis needs to be considered and ruled out when a patient with diabetes mellitus presents with a clinical picture of sinusitis. Diagnosis and treatment at this early stage will likely mean survival of the patient with minimal need for disfiguring surgery. If diagnosis is delayed and the disease progresses, the chances for a full recovery diminish significantly. Some patients with rhinocerebral mucormycosis present in diabetic ketoacidosis as the first time they were aware they had diabetes.

Diagnosis

The diagnosis of mucormycosis requires that tissue be examined for the presence of the characteristic irregular, broad, nonseptate, right-angle branching hyphae (Fig. 4). Since the organism invades tissue and blood vessels and may be found only scattered within a larger area of necrosis, superficial swabs are not sufficient to send to the laboratory for analysis. While scans and x-rays are not useful in establishing a definitive diagnosis, the presence of tissue destruction, especially traversing across anatomic boundaries should be a strong clue that mucormycosis may be the etiology of the problem. Thus, CT scans and MRI have been useful in defining the anatomic correlates of the infection. Extension of the pathology across tissue planes strongly suggests a fungal etiology and the need for biopsy in order to establish the diagnosis.

Treatment

Reversal of the underlying predisposing factors is a critical first step in the treatment of patients with mucormycosis. Thus, diabetic ketoacidosis needs to be aggressively managed, and doses of immunosuppressive drugs should be tapered and discontinued, if at all possible. Ampho-

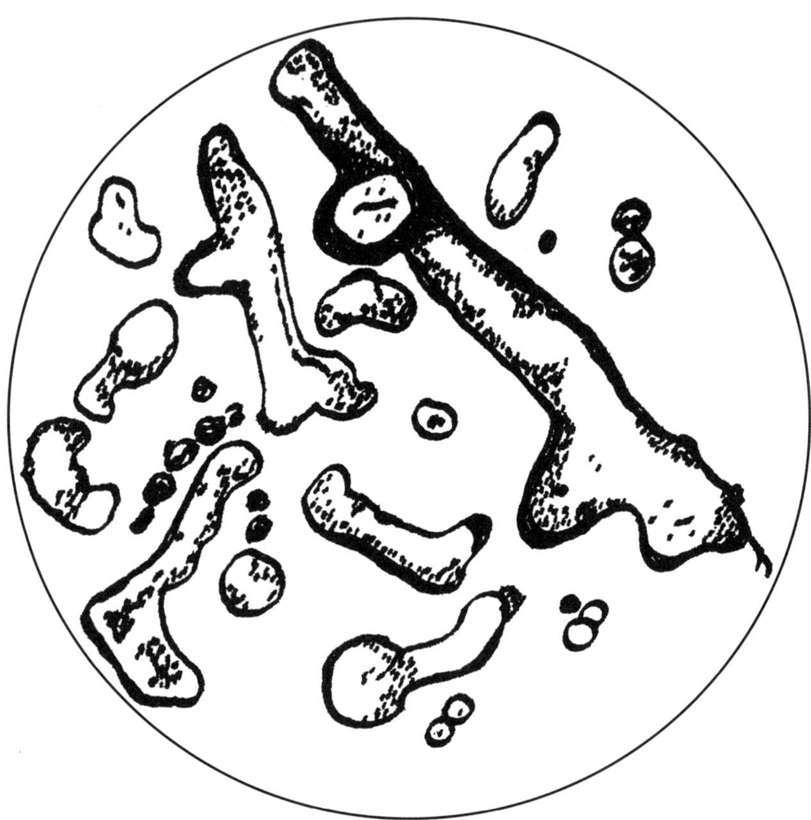

FIG. 4. Broad, irregular, pleomorphic, nonseptate hyphae with right-angle branching, suggestive of the fungi causing mucormycosis.

tericin B remains the drug of choice for the treatment of mucormycosis and should be given in high doses, 1 to 1.5 mg/kg/day, without the delay of increasing dose titration. Devitalized tissue needs to be removed and the best results seem to follow aggressive debridement, combined with high-dose amphotericin B. The role of hyperbaric oxygen has not been fully clarified, but can be used if facilities for the administration of high pressures of ambient oxygen are available.

THE DIMORPHIC FUNGI

The dimorphic fungi are so named because they exist in two distinct morphological forms (Table 8). In the environment, they produce hyphae and infectious conidia. At the elevated body temperature of humans and

TABLE 8. *The Dimorphic Fungi and Diseases They Cause*

Blastomyces dermatitidis	Blastomycosis
Coccidioides immitis	Coccidioidomycosis
Histoplasma capsulatum	Histoplasmosis
Paracoccidioides brasiliensis	Paracoccidioidomycosis
Sporothrix schenkii	Sporotrichosis

other animals, however, the conidia proliferate as yeast-like structures, which are able to overcome the defense mechanisms of the normal host. It is distinctly unusual to find hyphal elements of these fungi in infected tissue. In addition to their peculiar growth patterns, the dimorphic fungi are, with one exception, restricted by certain geographic considerations (Table 9). *Coccidioides immitis* is found in the arid areas of the American southwest and parts of Mexico and South America. *Histoplasma capsulatum* and *Blastomyces dermatitidis* are found in the Ohio and Mississippi river valleys, and *Paracoccidioides brasiliensis* is found throughout South America and certain islands of the Caribbean. The one dimorphic fungus that is cosmopolitan in its distribution is *Sporothrix schenkii*. Sporotrichosis is also different from the diseases caused by the other dimorphic fungi in that the route of infection is primarily through the skin and not via inhalation.

TABLE 9. *Geographic Regions Where Dimorphic Fungi Are Found**

Fungus	Endemic Region
Blastomyces dermatitidis	Ohio and Mississippi river valleys
Coccidioides immitis	Southwest United States, northern Mexico, parts of South America
Histoplasma capsulatum	Ohio and Mississippi river valleys, into northern Texas
Paracoccidioides brasiliensis	South and Central America
Sporothrix schenkii	Cosmopolitan

*With the ease of travel and the increase in the AIDS population, these organisms must be considered in other geographical locales.

9

Blastomyces Dermatitidis

Clinical

Blastomycosis is caused by the dimorphic fungus, *Blastomyces dermatitidis*. The organism presumably dwells in the soil in the endemic regions of the United States, which include the Midwest and extends along the U.S.-Canada border from the Great Lakes to the eastern coast. For reasons that are not understood, it has been extremely difficult to recover this fungus from the soil. However, outbreaks associated with the exposure of people to decaying wood in a moist environment have been reported. The disease is not contagious, but is acquired from the inhalation of conidia. The incubation period probably is 30 to 45 days.

Most people exposed to the organism remain asymptomatic. Some exposed individuals develop clinically evident pneumonia, which is most often self-limited. Symptoms include fever, chills, cough, sputum production, pleuritic chest pain, myalgias, and arthralgias. Exposure to a large inoculum can lead to the development of a rapidly progressive and potentially fatal pneumonia, with the development of adult respiratory distress syndrome. Dissemination beyond the lungs occurs in a small number of infected patients (approximately 5%) and most often involves the skin, bones, and prostate gland. Ten percent or less of patients with disseminated blastomycosis will develop mass lesions in the central nervous system.

Skin lesions may accompany active pulmonary infection, but can occur alone, as the sole manifestation of disseminated blastomycosis. Lesions may be wart-like, often originating as papulopustular, and eventually becoming crusted, lesions. Ulcerated skin lesions are also seen. In contrast to other cutaneous fungal infections, regional lymphadenopathy in these patients is unusual.

Some patients suffer from chronic pneumonia, which may present with cough, hemoptysis, chest pain, and weight loss. Chest x-rays are abnormal (see below).

Interestingly, in the immunosuppressed patient, blastomycosis is less common than coccidioidomycosis and histoplasmosis.

Diagnosis

Diagnosis is readily established following visualization of the organism in specimens. The characteristic doubly refractile cell wall and broad-based buds are unique features of *B. dermatitidis* (Fig. 5). The yeast is usually 8 to 15 µm in diameter. Sputum, biopsy specimens, and prostatic secretions may contain the fungus. Recovery of the fungus by culture of sputum or tissue biopsy samples is easily accomplished, with the yeast form of the organism growing readily at 30°C. Cultures should be held in the laboratory for 4 to 6 weeks prior to being reported as negative.

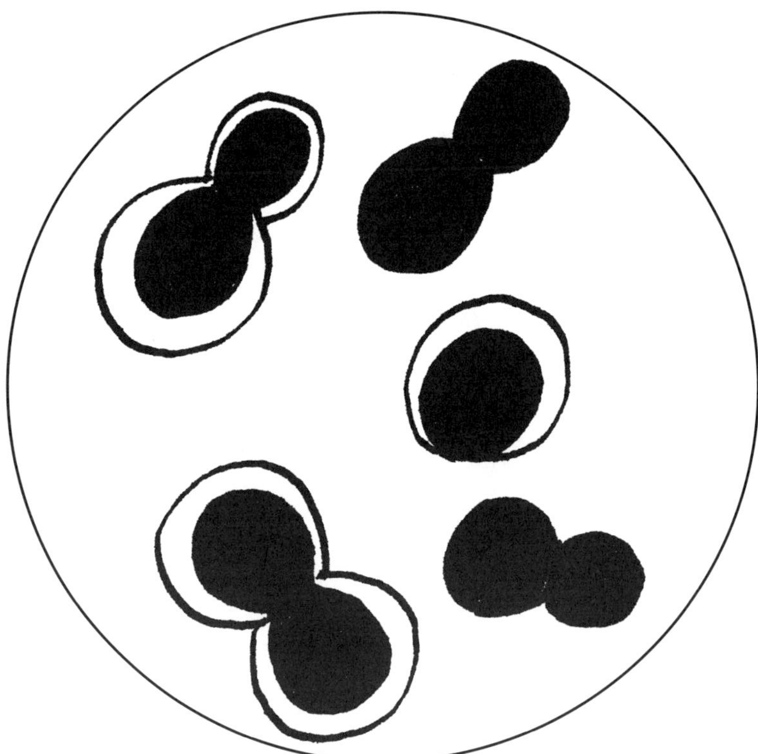

FIG. 5. Large yeast-like cell with single daughter bud. The yeast has thick, doubly refractile cell wall and wide connection to daughter bud, characteristic of *Blastomyces dermatitidis.*

Serologic assays are not yet clinically available, but there have been promising advances in the identification of a suitable diagnostic antigen.

Treatment

Patients with non-life-threatening disease are usually treated with an azole. Itraconazole, 200 to 400 mg/day, has replaced ketoconazole, due to its decreased toxicities and good efficacy. Fluconazole, in doses up to 400 mg/day, has not been as active and should not be used for initial therapy. In patients who experience life-threatening infection and in those with immunosuppression, many authorities would start treatment with amphotericin B, 0.8 to 1.2 mg/kg/day. Once the patient is stabilized and the infection better controlled, a switch to itraconazole can be made. Duration of therapy in pulmonary blastomycosis is usually about 6 months. Similar lengths of therapy are used for disseminated blastomycosis, but decisions about treatment duration need to be individualized and a longer course of therapy may be needed.

10

Coccidioides Immitis

Clinical

Coccidioidomycosis, "coccy" for short, has the unenviable reputation of being one of the most difficult mycoses to pronounce and spell in the English language. Often ignored in the differential diagnosis of illnesses outside of the endemic regions, this disease is capable of mimicking many different diseases, including malignancies, pneumonia, meningitis, abscesses, and osteomyelitis. Thus, practitioners in the endemic areas become adept at recognizing the varied presentations of "coccy."

Known as "valley fever," its name comes from the presence of the causative fungus *Coccidioides immitis,* in the soil of the desert areas of southern California, especially the San Joaquin Valley. However, the range of "coccy country" extends through Arizona into northern and central Mexico. Coccidioidomycosis was discovered in 1873 by Posadas, a third-year medical student in Argentina. Cases have been reported from most countries of South America.

Most people exposed to the fungus do not become ill. However, approximatcly 50% of infected patients experience a nonspecific flu-like illness characterized by fever, myalgias, headache, dry cough, and pleuritic chest pain. In a much smaller number of patients, <10%, dissemination to extrapulmonary locations occurs. Most commonly, skin, bones, and meninges are involved when dissemination occurs.

The most common clinically recognizable illness due to infection with *C. immitis* is "valley fever," which is characterized by the development of fever, arthralgias, arthritis, and erythema multiforme or erythema nodosum. The latter cutaneous manifestation is thought to be an allergic phenomenon, is indicative of a good prognosis, and does not contain the fungus. In addition, erythema nodosum occurs primarily in women.

The clinical manifestations of disseminated coccidioidomycosis depend on which organs are involved. For example, cutaneous coccidioidomycosis presents with a variety of skin lesions, which on culture contain the fungus. Papules, pustules, ulcers, and nodular lesions have been described. Subcutaneous abscesses also occur, as do fistulas connecting skin with deeper structures.

Bone and joint coccidioidomycosis involves long bones and vertebrae preferentially, although almost any bone in the body can be infected. About 40% of patients have more than one bone involved. Destruction of the vertebrae is particularly ominous, as spinal cord compromise can readily follow destabilization of the spine. Differential diagnosis includes tuberculosis, brucellosis, other infectious causes of osteomyelitis, and tumors.

Coccidioidal meningitis is most commonly seen in white men. Without treatment, this is a fatal disease, with most patients dying within 2 years of diagnosis. Patients present with headache, mental status or personality changes, and symptoms of increased intracranial pressure, such as nausea and vomiting. Fever usually occurs, but less than half of patients will complain of stiff neck or have signs of meningismus. Meningitis can occur within a month of exposure to the fungus in soil, but presentation may be delayed for over 1 year. Thus, a careful review of the travel history is needed in order to suspect this diagnosis.

Diagnosis

Diagnosis depends on the identification of the fungus, either by microscopy or culture. Direct examination of sputum, CSF, exudates, or tissue, using KOH or calcofluor, is recommended over examination of culture due to the highly infectious nature of the filamentous form of the organism. The characteristic spherules of *C. immitis* are thick-walled, 20 to 60 μm in diameter (Fig. 6). If intact, they will contain endospores, 2 to 4 μm in diameter, or if disrupted, the endospores will be seen surrounding the spherule. Histologically, the fungus also is visualized easily in GMS, PAS, or H&E stained specimens.

Treatment

The treatment of all manifestations of coccidioidomycosis has been revolutionized with the introduction of the azole antifungals into clinical practice. Amphotericin B is currently reserved for patients with severe, progressive, life-threatening infection, which often includes many immunocompromised patients. Otherwise, therapy can begin with

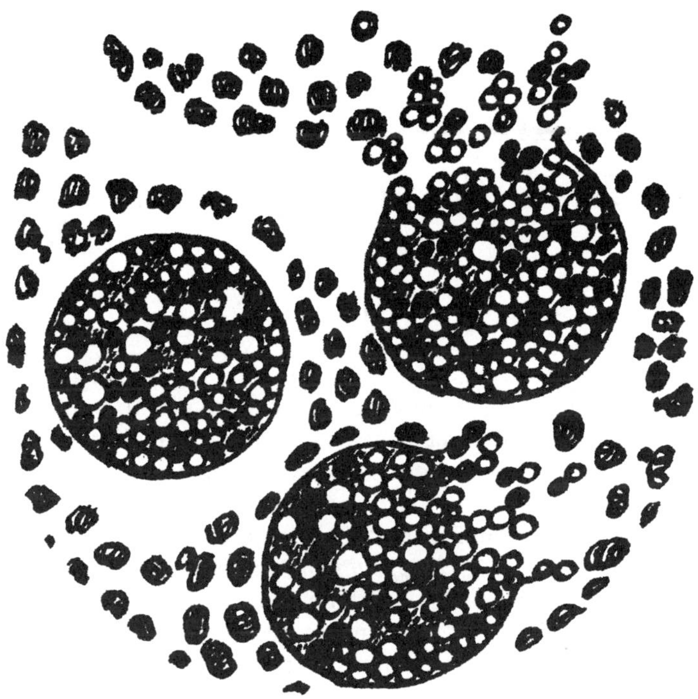

FIG. 6. Large spherule containing innumerable endospores, characteristic of *Coccidioides immitis.*

an azole. Ketoconazole has been used quite successfully for years, but itraconazole has replaced ketoconazole for most indications, because it is better tolerated. The usual dose of itraconazole for all manifestations of coccidioidomycosis is 200 mg twice daily.

One exception to this recommendation is the treatment of coccidioidal meningitis, which is now treated with fluconazole, 800 to 1,200 mg/day. Since patients have relapsed once therapy is discontinued, most authorities now recommend life-long fluconazole therapy in these patients. In critically ill patients, intrathecal amphotericin B is still used, but long-term therapy with this route of administration of amphotericin B has now been replaced with high-dose fluconazole. Should intrathecal amphotericin B be required, consultation with experts in the treatment of coccidioidal meningitis should be obtained.

11

Histoplasma capsulatum

Clinical

This disease follows inhalation of microconidia produced by *Histoplasma capsulatum*. The fungus grows as hyphae in soil, especially that enriched by bird or bat droppings, in specific geographic areas, including the Ohio and Mississippi river valleys, along the U.S.-Canada border from the Great Lakes to the eastern coast, into eastern Texas, and to some areas in northern Florida. Foci can also be found in areas of Africa. A second species, *H. capsulatum* var. *duboisii* is found in tropical areas of Africa and causes a different type of disease than the histoplasmosis caused by the more common *H. capsulatum*. Further details can be found in standard medical mycology texts.

Following inhalation of the fungus, most people (probably 90%) remain asymptomatic. Primary pulmonary histoplasmosis is the main manifestation in those who develop symptoms. The illness develops 3 days to 3 weeks after exposure, and patients complain of nonspecific systemic symptoms such as fever, chills, headache, chest pain, malaise, and myalgias. About 5% of patients, mostly women, will develop joint pains, arthritis, erythema nodosum, or erythema multiforme. Other rare manifestations of acute histoplasmosis are pericarditis and adult respiratory distress syndrome (ARDS). This latter manifestation may develop after unusually heavy exposures.

Lung involvement also can be subacute to chronic, with the presence of one or more nodules, representing a discrete focus of the organisms, known as a histoplasmoma. These are indistinguishable from "coin lesions," and usually need to be diagnosed following biopsy. It is common for patients with histoplasmosis to develop hilar and mediastinal lymphadenopathy. Occasionally, as the lesions resolve, a brisk fibrotic reaction can occur, resulting in mediastinal fibrosis. This process can be progressive and unremitting, resulting in superior vena cava syndrome and other complications resulting from constriction of mediastinal structures.

Chronic pulmonary histoplasmosis closely mimics pulmonary tuberculosis in appearance and symptomatology. A majority of patients are elderly men with chronic obstructive pulmonary disease. Persistent cough, anorexia, weight loss, and fever are common complaints.

The fungus may disseminate beyond the lungs to other organs. Manifestations can occur with the primary pulmonary infection or become evident years later. Immunocompromised patients, including those with AIDS, frequently develop acute progressive disseminated histoplasmosis. This form of the disease also occurs in infants and young children and those taking immunosuppressive drugs. Patients typically are febrile and complain of weight loss, malaise, cough, and dyspnea. Meningitis will develop in less than 20% of AIDS patients with this form of the fungal disease.

Diagnosis

Definitive diagnosis of histoplasmosis is established by identifying the organism in sputum, other fluids, or tissue obtained by biopsy. Direct examination of specimens using KOH or calcofluor are less reliable than for the other dimorphic fungi. The small unicellular budding yeast may not be reliably detected because of their size (2 to 5 μm) or may be confused with *Candida* (*Torulopsis*) *glabrata,* which is similar in size and shape (Fig. 7). The organism is frequently seen within the cytoplasm of macrophages, which is clearly visible in H&E or PAS stained specimens. The organism elicits a granulomatous inflammatory response, which can be seen histologically. *H. capsulatum* may be confused with other intracellular parasites, such as *Leishmania donovani* or *Toxoplasma gondii. Pneumocystis carinii* are slightly larger (5 to 8 μm), are extracellular and do not bud, which are important differential diagnostic features.

Cultures of specimens should be held for up to 6 weeks when the diagnosis is suspected, because *H. capsulatum* grows very slowly in culture. Macroscopically, it grows as a white to buff colony, but microscopically, it produces characteristic tuberculate and nontuberculate macroconidia. *Sepedonium,* a saprophytic organism, produces similar macroconidia, thus making further analysis necessary for definitive identification, such as conversion of the filamentous form to the yeast form or a positive reaction with a specific nucleic acid probe.

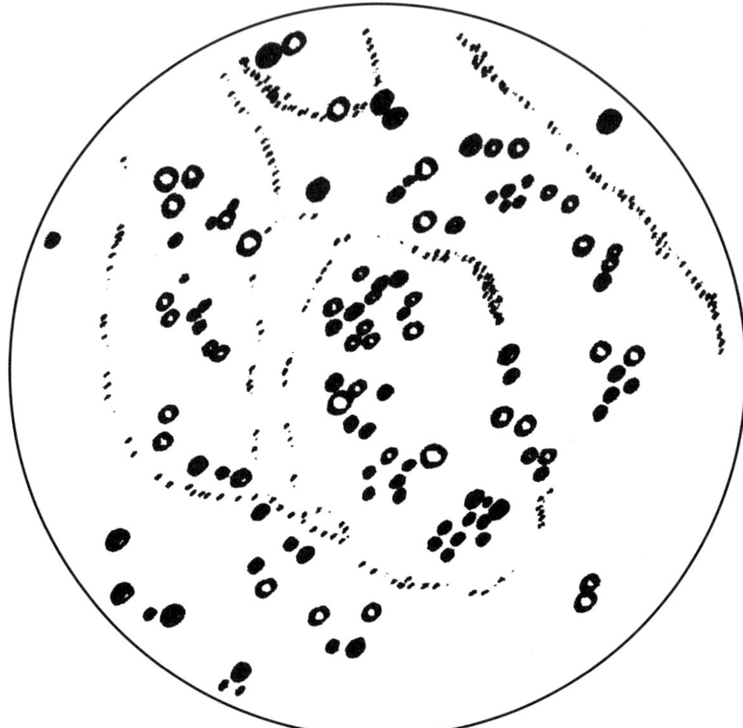

FIG. 7. Small budding yeasts, no hyphae or pseudohyphae, most compatible with *Histoplasma capsulatum, Candida* (*Torulopsis*) *glabrata.* On silver-stained sections can be confused with *Pneumocystis carinii.*

The chest x-ray is abnormal in patients with acute pulmonary histoplasmosis. Lesions may be focal or diffuse, and cavitation may be observed. In the most seriously ill, a miliary pattern can be seen. Hilar and mediastinal adenopathy may be present. Laboratory testing provides nonspecific results. One interesting presentation is that of diffuse pulmonary calcifications ("popcorn" calcifications), which represent healed pulmonary histoplasmosis. These patients are totally asymptomatic and need no treatment for this inactive remnant of the acute infection.

Histoplasmosis skin testing is not recommended since a positive test only suggests previous exposure to the fungus, but not active infection. Antibody tests are available and are often useful in confirming the diagnosis. Complement fixing (CF) antibodies (IgG) in titers ≥ 1:8 are considered positive. Titers of at least 1:32 are suggestive of acute histoplasmosis. Seroconversion can be demonstrated by testing sera obtained 4 to 6 weeks after the patient presents for care. By this time, up to 95%

of patients will have positive titers. In patients with chronic histoplasmosis, CF titers can remain elevated for years. In others, however, the titers fall with time.

Immunodiffusion (ID) tests using two mycelia-derived antigens, H and M, also may be useful in making the diagnosis. Within four weeks of exposure to the fungus, up to 80% of patients demonstrate a positive ID reaction to M antigen. These antibodies tend to persist for years and can cross react with antigens from the other dimorphic fungi. In contrast, ID reactions to the H antigen occur only in approximately 20% of patients with acute histoplasmosis, are usually present for only up to 6 months after the acute infection, and are less cross reactive with other fungal antigens. Therefore, a positive test for antibodies to H antigen is more specific for active histoplasmosis.

Antigen testing for a polysaccharide antigen in blood, urine, or cerebrospinal fluid is available through the Histoplasmosis Reference Laboratory (Appendix 20) and is useful in confirming the diagnosis of active histoplasmosis as well as following response to therapy, especially in AIDS patients. Successfully treated patients show a drop in the antigen titers—an increase in titer portends relapse or breakthrough if the patient is being treated. Detection of the polysaccharide antigen is less sensitive in non-HIV-infected patients with localized pulmonary disease.

Treatment

The drug of choice for most critically ill patients with acute histoplasmosis is amphotericin B. Doses of 0.7 to 1.0 mg/kg/day are typically administered for several weeks, until the patient has stabilized and the acute infection has been controlled. Then a switch to itraconazole, 200 mg twice daily, is often used, replacing ketoconazole, which was formerly the azole of choice. If there is no underlying immunosuppression, a 2- to 3-month regimen may be all that is required. However, in patients with persistent immunosuppression, such as those with AIDS, life-long therapy will be required, and the differentiation between primary and then consolidation or maintenance therapy is sometimes unclear. Maintenance therapy in the AIDS patient is considered chronic suppressive therapy and is best achieved with itraconazole, 200 mg twice daily for life.

Ketoconazole has been used in the treatment of acute histoplasmosis, but has been largely replaced by the better tolerated itraconazole. Fluconazole in doses $\leq$ 400 mg daily have been somewhat less effective than itraconazole in treating histoplasmosis. Trials evaluating higher doses of fluconazole are underway.

Patients with histoplasmosis meningitis or endocarditis are usually treated with amphotericin B for many months. Surgical removal of the infected heart valve is usually important adjunctive therapy. The role of chronic itraconazole therapy is unclear, but it seems reasonable to consider it in carefully selected patients. Isolated histoplasmomas requires no specific antifungal therapy. Other focal infections, such as bone or joint, skin, and other isolated areas of involvement can be treated with itraconazole, 200 mg twice daily, for variable periods, but usually over many months, until all evidence of active infection is gone.

The treatment of mediastinal fibrosis is difficult and controversial. With the availability of azoles that can be safely administered for long periods, it seems reasonable to treat with itraconazole for months (perhaps up to 6 months or longer) in an attempt to eradicate any remaining viable fungi. No benefits appear from the use of corticosteroids, and the role of other drugs, such as the newer immunomodulators, is yet unknown.

12

Paracoccidioides Brasiliensis

Clinical

Paracoccidioidomycosis occurs primarily in patients from South America. The causative agent, *Paracoccidioides brasiliensis*, is an airborne pathogen. Although its precise source in the environment is not known definitively, it is thought to reside in the soil. Because estrogen inhibits the conversion of the mycelia form to the yeast-like form, men predominate with this disease by a ratio of 16:1. Most patients present with pulmonary complaints, but dissemination to other areas of the body can occur, including bone, meninges, skin, and abdominal organs.

Tuberculosis can coexist with paracoccidioidomycosis in up to 25% of patients; therefore, all patients with paracoccidioidomycosis need to be evaluated for this infection as well.

Diagnosis

Most patients who are producing sputum or in whom exudates can be obtained will have the organism in those samples. A direct examination with KOH or calcofluor will reveal the characteristic large (4 to 40 μm), multiply budding yeast forms (Fig. 8). The same appearance is found on histologic slides stained with GMS or PAS. The yeasts often are found in the presence of a mixed neutrophilic-granulomatous inflammatory response.

Paracoccidioides brasiliensis may take 4 to 6 weeks to grow from specimens submitted to the laboratory, but a positive culture is definitive proof of the etiologic agent responsible for the infectious process.

Serology is also a useful adjunct for making the diagnosis and following the progress of therapy. Most patients will develop antibodies that can be detected by an immunodiffusion (ID) test. This test is highly

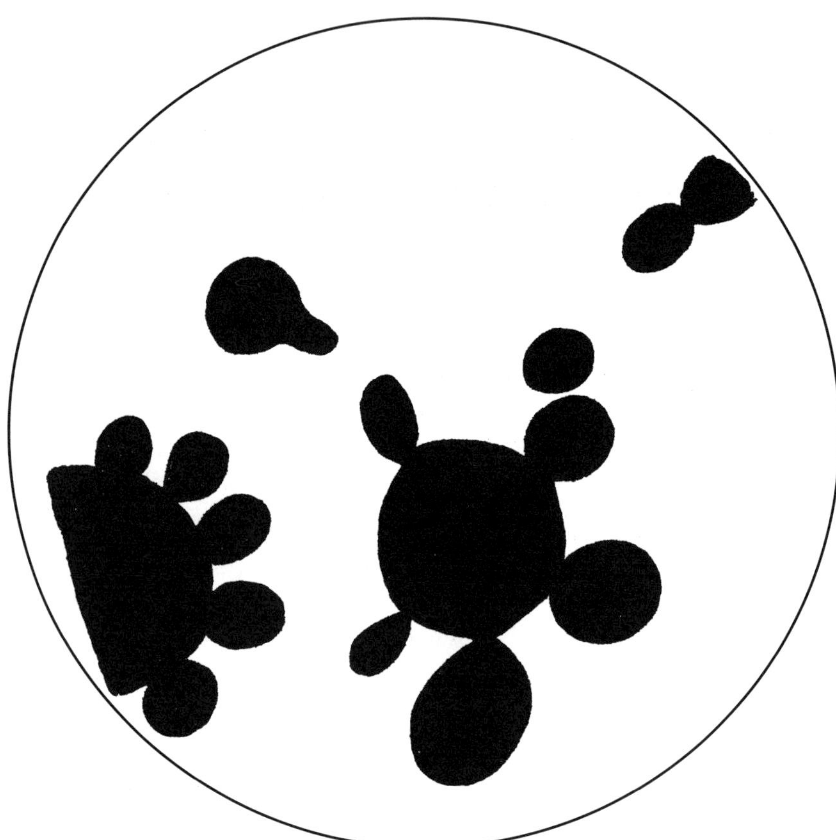

FIG. 8. Yeast-like cell with multiple budding daughter cells, often in the shape of a "pilot's wheel." Characteristic of *Paracoccidioides brasiliensis.*

specific and the presence of antibodies to precipitin bands 1 and 2 is diagnostic. A complement fixation (CF) test is also available, but cross reactions with *Histoplasma capsulatum* confound interpretation of the results. Enzyme-based assays have also been proposed for use in diagnosis, but may not be widely available. A newly developed DNA probe may be useful for rapid DNA-based diagnostic tests. Skin testing is not used to make the diagnosis of paracoccidioidomycosis.

Treatment

Historically, paracoccidioidomycosis was treated with sulfonamides; however, with the advent of azoles, the sulfonamides are used rarely now, since long-term therapy (i.e., years) is often required. Ketoconazole has been very effective in controlling symptoms, but itraconazole has supplanted ketoconazole, in large part due to safety issues: Itraconazole has less toxicity than ketoconazole.

Since most patients with this disease are from poorer areas of the world, cost is an important consideration when treating patients, who may require many months of therapy to insure cure. Itraconazole, 100 mg daily, results in good clinical responses and a low rate of relapse (<5%).

13

Sporothrix Schenckii

Clinical

Sporothrix schenkii is a dimorphic fungus, found throughout the world. In contrast to the other dimorphic fungi, this organism usually causes disease following percutaneous inoculation rather than following inhalation. Thus, the most common presentations involve the skin and not the lungs. However, in the severely immunocompromised host and in patients with AIDS, disseminated sporotrichosis has been reported. The typical patient has been exposed to the organism from contact with soil or decaying wood. The classic predisposing avocation is rose gardening, probably because of the sphagnum peat moss used in growing these plants. Some trauma, which may be relatively minor and difficult to recall, may be reported.

The lesions begin as papular lesions, evolving into pustular and ulcerated lesions. Typically, a chain of lesions develops as the disease progresses, giving rise to the term "sporotrichoid" appearance. Other organisms, such as *Nocardia,* and atypical *Mycobacteria,* especially *M. marinum* and *M. kansasii,* can present in this way. Single lesions also can be confused with cutaneous leishmaniasis, blastomycosis, chromoblastomycosis, and cutaneous tuberculosis.

Disseminated sporotrichosis also may occur, most commonly involving joints. Occasionally, pulmonary sporotrichosis is found, usually in alcoholics or those with other medical illnesses, such as diabetes mellitus, sarcoidosis, or tuberculosis. Chronic corticosteroid use also may be a predisposing factor. Lung involvement is characterized by unilateral or bilateral cavitation, with or without infiltrate. A rare manifestation of sporotrichosis is chronic meningitis, which presents as a chronic lymphocytic meningitis.

Diagnosis

In skin lesions, the fungus may be difficult to detect because of relatively low numbers of organisms present in the lesions. When visible, the yeasts are small (3 to 5 μm) and oval to cigar shaped (Fig. 9). Histologically, asteroid bodies, which consist of a yeast-like, somewhat basophilic center (3 to 5μm in diameter), with a radiating eosinophilic border (approximately 10μm thick), may be present. These may be seen with coccidioidomycosis and aspergillosis as well, so they are not diagnostic for sporotrichosis. Cultures also may be negative due to low number of organisms, and repeated biopsies may be needed to confirm the diagnosis. Mixed neutrophilic and granulomatous inflammation may be present.

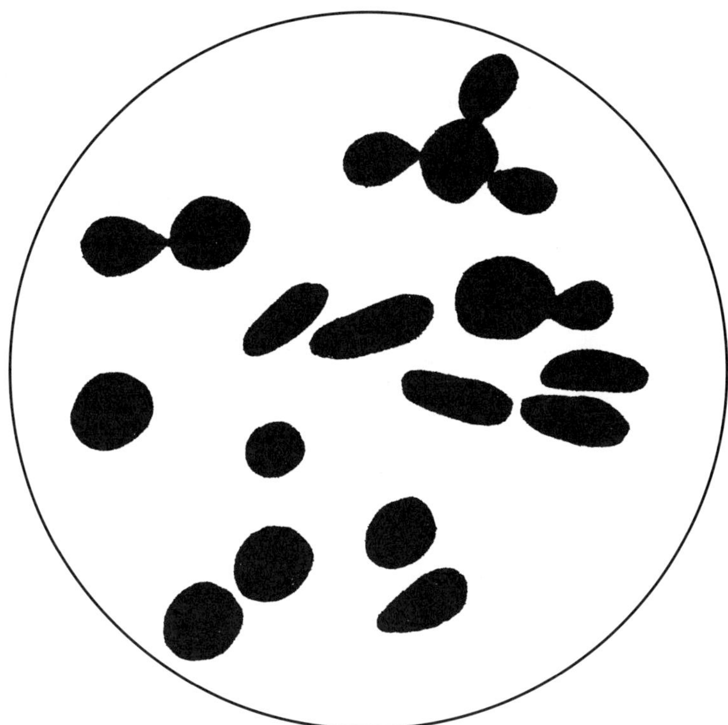

FIG. 9. Yeasts of *Sporothrix schenkii.* Usually, not many of the characteristic oval to cigar-shaped yeasts are present in any given section.

Treatment

The greatest experience in treatment of sporotrichosis is with supersaturated potassium iodide (SSKI). SSKI is prescribed by the drop. Therapy is started with five to ten drops, three times daily. The dose is gradually increased to 25 to 40 drops, three times daily, in children; 40 to 50 drops, three times daily, in adults. This drug has a bitter taste and must be given in some liquid in order to mask the flavor. Typical side effects with iodide are nausea, vomiting, diarrhea, salivary and lachrymal gland enlargement, and acneiform rash. Therapy must be administered for approximately 2 to 3 months, until the skin lesions have resolved. Because this therapy is relatively well tolerated and is quite inexpensive, many use iodides as the drug of choice in treating lymphocutaneous sporotrichosis. In patients intolerant of iodides, itraconazole, 100 to 200 mg bid, has been used with good success and has largely replaced ketoconazole. Fluconazole, in doses $\leq$ 400 mg/day, appears to be less effective than itraconazole.

Noncutaneous forms of sporotrichosis are more difficult to treat. Amphotericin B may need to be used initially in critically ill patients, but itraconazole, 200 mg bid, is preferred in those whose disease is not life-threatening. The treatment of *S. schenkii* meningitis is very difficult and amphotericin B plus flucytosine may be the best therapy. There is very little experience with the azoles in this less-common presentation of the disease.

14

Unusual Fungi Causing Disease

PENICILLIUM MARNEFFEI

Clinical

This dimorphic fungus causes disease primarily in patients infected with HIV, but infections in non-HIV infected people are also well described. The disease has been relatively rare in the United States, however, since the fungus is endemic in southeast Asia. Bamboo rats are also infected by the fungus and may play a role in its life cycle. Infection is characterized by involvement of the reticuloendothelial system and can closely mimic disseminated histoplasmosis. Most patients will have fever and chills and respiratory complaints such as cough, dyspnea, and chest pain; malaise and weight loss are common. Lymph nodes, liver and spleen are enlarged in approximately 40% of patients. Skin lesions are present more frequently than in histoplasmosis, and are papular, ulcerated, or acneiform in appearance. The fungus can also produce mulloscum contagiosum-like lesions.

Diagnosis

Microscopic examination of smears or histopathological slides is a rapid way to make a presumptive diagnosis. The fungus replicates by fission, with internal septations of the round to oval cells (Fig. 10). Budding is not seen. The fungal elements are often found inside macrophages. The fungus grows in soil in the mycelial phase and in tissue in a yeast-like form. Anemia may be present, but is a nonspecific finding.

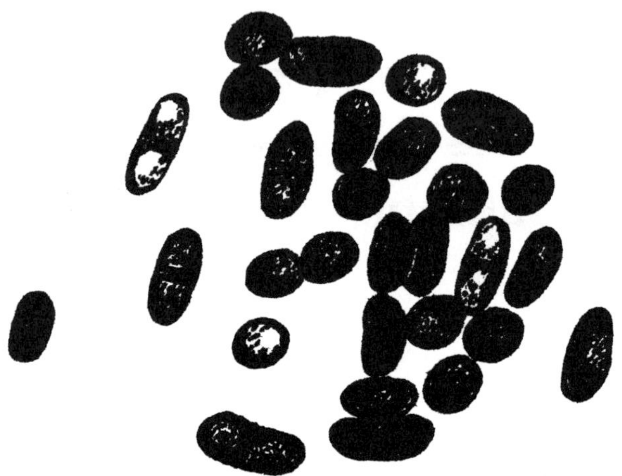

FIG. 10. Characteristic oval, sausage-shaped yeast-like cells with internal septae characteristic of *Penicillium marneffei.*

Treatment

Without therapy, disseminated penicilliosis is a fatal disease. Therapy, however, is difficult, since responses to available agents are not optimal. The initial induction course of treatment is often with amphotericin B, 1 mg/kg/day, and flucytosine, 100 to 150 mg/kg/day. Once the patient has improved, switching to an azole is possible—itraconazole has been used most frequently for treatment of this infection. In the AIDS patient, therapy should continue for life. Duration of treatment in non-AIDS patients is unknown, but should probably last for at least 1 year.

TRICHOSPORON SPECIES

Clinical

Trichosporon beigelii, the etiologic agent of white piedra (a superficial infection of the hair shaft) in immunocompetent hosts, has emerged as an infrequent but often fatal opportunistic fungal pathogen in immunocompromised patients. The most common predisposing factors for disseminated *Trichosporon* infections are granulocytopenia and corticosteroid therapy, but the disease has also been associated with organ transplantation, hemochromatosis, prosthetic valve surgery, and possibly AIDS. Clinical manifestations mimic those of disseminated candidiasis, including fever, refractory fungemia, hematuria, cutaneous lesions, chorioretinitis, pulmonary infiltrates, and renal failure. The cutaneous lesions occur frequently beginning as erythematous papules, which evolve into maculonodular erythematous lesions, frequently developing central necrosis or forming hemorrhagic bullae.

Diagnosis

While the cutaneous lesions occur frequently, they are not pathognomonic for *Trichosporon* infections. If the three morphologic forms of the fungus (blastoconidia, arthroconidia, and hyphae) are visible histologically, a diagnosis of trichosporonosis may be made. Otherwise, a positive culture is necessary to differentiate these lesions from those caused by *Candida* spp., *Fusarium* spp., *Pseudallescheria* spp., or *Aspergillus* spp. The organism is easily recovered from blood, urine, and tissue. Once isolated, the yeast can be identified by standard biochemical profiles.

Chest x-rays may reveal lobar consolidation, bronchopneumonia, or a reticulonodular pattern, all of which are nonspecific findings.

Sera from patients with disseminated *Trichosporon* infections have been shown to have positive latex agglutination tests for *C. neoformans.* While nonencapsulated, *T. beigelii* shares antigenic determinants with the polysaccharide component glucoronoxylomannan of *C. neoformans.* This antigen may play a role in modulating host defense against *T. beigelii,* which may contribute to the poor prognosis in patients with disseminated trichosporonosis.

Treatment

Many cases of trichosporonosis have been reported to be refractory to amphotericin B therapy. A combination of amphotericin B (1 to 1.5 mg/kg/day) plus flucytosine (50 to 100 mg/kg/day) has been used with some success. Fluconazole, 400 to 1,200 mg/day, which has good activity against the organism, also has been used with success and may be the drug of choice for this disease. Reversal of the underlying immunosuppression may be the most important factor in the survival of patients with disseminated *Trichosporon* infections. Recent *in vitro* studies have demonstrated that GM-CSF, M-CSF, and IFN-γ augment antifungal activity of peripheral blood mononuclear cells, suggesting the need for further evaluation of these cytokines as potential adjunct therapy.

MALASSEZIA FURFUR (PITYROSPORUM OVALE)

Clinical

This organism is a member of the normal human cutaneous flora. It may be associated with chronic superficial fungal disease, folliculitis, atopic dermatitis; unlike other dermatophytic organisms, it also may cause systemic disease. *Malassezia furfur* is a lipophilic organism and as such, systemic disease primarily has been associated with intravenous lipid alimentation. It may cause a catheter-related fungemia, especially in newborn infants receiving lipid-supplemented total parenteral nutrition. The clinical manifestations include fungemia, thrombocytopenia, and respiratory distress.

Another *Malassezia* spp., *M. pachydermitis*, also has been associated with systemic disease similar in presentation to that of *M. furfur*, but has not been associated with fatty acid supplementation.

Diagnosis

Examination of blood smears drawn through the catheter may reveal the globose, oblong to cylindrical yeast cells characteristic of *M. furfur*. If *M. furfur* is suspected as the cause of fungemia, the microbiology laboratory should be notified in advance so that blood cultures may be supplemented with olive oil to increase the likelihood of recovering the organism.

Treatment

Successful treatment of this disease requires discontinuation of the lipid infusion and removal of the venous catheter. Fluconazole, 400 mg daily, is the drug of choice for intravenous administration, while fluconazole or itraconazole may be administered orally in the more stable patients. Amphotericin B has been ineffective in treating patients with this infection.

AGENTS CAUSING PHAEOHYPHOMYCOSIS

Clinical

Phaeohyphomycoses are deep tissue infections caused by the dematiaceous fungi. Some of these include *Cladosporium bantianum, Wang-*

iella dermatitidis, Bipolaris spp., and *P. boydii.* Infection due to *C. bantianum* can occur in patients with no apparent immunosuppression, and is often fatal due to the high propensity of this organism to invade the central nervous system. Like *C. bantianum, W. dermatitidis* is also neurotropic and thus has been implicated in CNS infections, as well as its more common role as a causative agent of mycetoma. *Bipolaris* spp. are common causes of phaeomycotic sinusitis, keratitis, and peritonitis in patients on continuous ambulatory peritoneal dialysis.

Clinical manifestations of disease are similar among these fungi and depend primarily on the location of the infection. Presentations are dependent on the specific site involved and the extent of the infection.

Diagnosis

The fungi causing the various systemic diseases described above can be presumptively identified by virtue of the melanin in their cell walls. The dark cell walls may be visible on KOH preparations or on hematoxylin- and eosin-stained tissue sections. However, melanin production may not be as great on occasion and in this case, the hyphae may be difficult to see unless silver or PAS stains are used as with other fungi. Biopsy of the involved area is critical so that the organism can be grown in the laboratory.

Treatment

Therapy is usually a combined medical and surgical effort. If foreign bodies are in place, they should be removed, if possible. Solitary lesions, such as in the brain or on skin, can be excised. The role of adjunctive antifungal therapy in these cases is unclear, especially since the intrinsic activity of available antifungal drugs does not appear to be very great. However, it seems worthwhile, especially with invasive disease of the CNS, to treat with amphotericin B, 1 mg/kg/day, as tolerated, to assess response of residual disease or other foci of infection. Liposomal amphotericin B preparations may be particularly attractive in this setting, given their relative safety and the need for long-term treatment of these invasive lesions. The role of azoles is unclear, but itraconazole, given its apparent broader spectrum of action against molds than the other azoles, may prove to be useful in this setting. Careful monitoring of the patient being treated with such an oral azole regimen is critical. This includes measuring itraconazole serum concentrations to ensure absorption.

PART 3

Principles of Antifungal Therapy

15

Introduction

The field of antifungal chemotherapy is relatively new; amphotericin B was introduced into clinical practice in 1958 (Table 10). For years, amphotericin B was the only reliable therapy for fungal diseases and thus, virtually by default, it became the gold standard for antifungal therapy of invasive mycoses. Subsequently, new drugs have been made available only sporadically. Flucytosine, which in the early 1960s was found to have antifungal activity, was initially tried as a single agent, but the rapid development of resistance and its limited spectrum of activity severely curtailed its use. The first two azoles developed for human use were both imidazoles: miconazole and clotrimazole. They both have been associated with numerous toxicities when administered intravenously, and thus, they now are used almost exclusively as topical antifungal agents.

The introduction of ketoconazole in 1979, however, marked a real change in our ability to treat invasive fungal infections for chronic mycoses such as coccidioidomycosis and the other endemic mycoses. The drug had a relatively low toxicity profile when compared to amphotericin B, but it soon became clear that doses of greater than 400 mg/day were often associated with unacceptable endocrinologic side effects.

Fluconazole was introduced in the 1980s when the AIDS epidemic caused an exponential increase in the number of severely immunocompromised patients. In addition to mucosal candidiasis, a number of these patients were becoming infected with fungi causing invasive disease. Studies demonstrated that fluconazole could be useful as primary therapy for many of these infections, but its major impact has been on long-term suppressive (maintenance) therapy of mucosal candidiasis and cryptococcosis. Initially, low doses of fluconazole (e.g., 50 to 100 mg/day) very often were effective in the treatment of thrush and were routinely used, especially by patients in Europe. Shortly after the explosion of use of fluconazole in AIDS patients, reports of the development

TABLE 10. *Antifungal Drugs Available for Use in Clinical Practice to Treat Invasive Fungal Infections*

Antifungal Drug	Year Approved for Use in USA
Amphotericin B (Fungizone®)	1958
Flucytosine	1957
Miconazole	1971
Ketoconazole	1983
Fluconazole	1990
Itraconazole	1994
Amphotericin B Lipid Complex (ABLC)	1995
Amphotericin B Colloidal Dispersion (ABCD)	1996

of resistance appeared. Studies now indicate a fairly complicated series of events that can culminate in decreased clinical responsiveness of patients to fluconazole (discussed in Chapter 18).

The most recently introduced orally administered azole derivative is itraconazole. This drug is the first oral agent active against molds and, in particular, *Aspergillus* spp. While serious issues surround the proper environment for the oral administration of itraconazole, this drug has provided a possible alternative to amphotericin B in treating invasive aspergillosis.

Several new drugs, including new azole agents, are under development (reviewed briefly in Chapter 19). These drugs promise to have broader spectra of activity than currently available agents, to be less toxic, to perhaps have fewer drug interactions, to be useful in antifungal drug combinations, and to have the versatility of oral and intravenous formulations.

16

The Polyenes: Amphotericin B and Nystatin

AMPHOTERICIN B

Despite the introduction of newer antifungal drugs, amphotericin B remains the primary antifungal drug for use in patients critically ill with an invasive mycosis. It is available for intravenous injection as Fungizone® and as generic amphotericin B. Amphotericin B is a polyene antifungal drug and is insoluble in water (Fig. 11). The commercial preparation is a micellar suspension in deoxycholate. Recently, liposomal formulations have been developed and FDA approval for each has occurred (amphotericin B lipid complex, ABCD) or will soon be finalized (AmBisome, Table 11). The role for conventional amphotericin B is well defined, but the niche for the liposomal preparations remains to be established.

Amphotericin B binds avidly to ergosterol, a major sterol component of the fungal, but not human, cell membrane. Low concentrations result in permeabilization of the cell with leakage of intracellular contents, most commonly measured as a loss in intracellular potassium. Higher concentrations lead to cell death. The drug can also bind, although with less affinity, to other sterols such as cholesterol, the major sterol in mammalian cell membranes. Despite the preferential binding of amphotericin B to ergosterol over cholesterol, much of the toxicity seen with amphotericin B is thought to arise from this interaction with human cells. By liposome encapsulation or associating the drug with lipids, it is hoped that efficacy may be preserved and toxicity can be minimized. Clearly, liposome formulations are much less toxic than conventional amphotericin B, and preliminary indications suggest that efficacy is not diminished. However, definitive proof of therapeutic equivalence may never be rigorously established given the many problems with satisfactory study design and patient accrual.

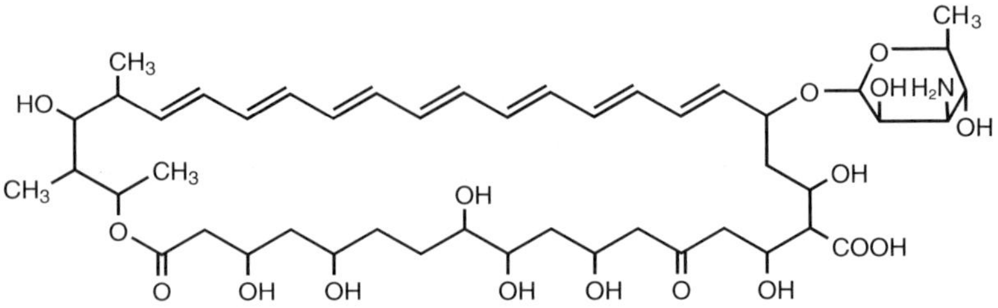

Amphotericin B

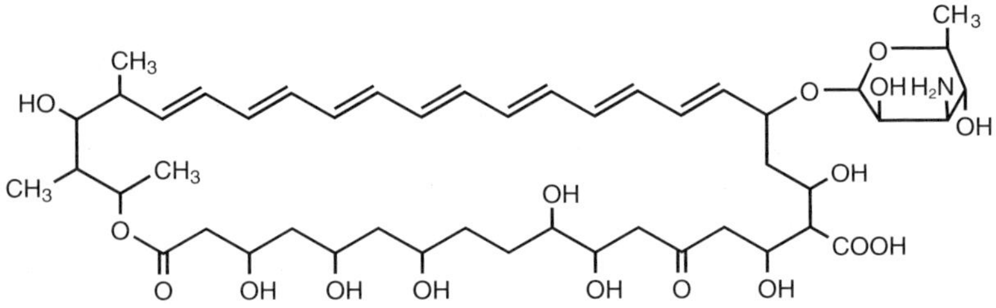

Nystatin

FIG. 11. Structure of the polyenes amphotericin B and nystatin.

Following an intravenous injection of conventional amphotericin B, serum concentrations fall below 1 μg/ml within 30 to 60 minutes. The drug is highly lipoprotein-bound and distributes into lipophilic tissues. When measured in the liver, for example, very high concentrations of amphotericin B can be measured by HPLC (>1,000 μg/ml). However, when measured by bioassay, very little if any amphotericin B can be detected. One explanation for this is the competition of lipids and sterols in the liver with fungal cells for the amphotericin B. The clinical relevance of this observation is unclear, but may be responsible for modulation of amphotericin B effects. The best clinical example of this phenomenon is the poor track record of amphotericin B in the treatment of hepatosplenic candidiasis.

Amphotericin B is not metabolized, but accumulates in lipid-rich tissues throughout the body. For up to several months, small amounts of amphotericin B are excreted into the urine and small amounts also appear in the bile. Presumably, amphotericin B, which concentrates in

TABLE 11. *Lipid Formulations of Amphotericin B*

Name	Company	Composition	Structure
ABLC (Abelcet®)	The Liposome Company	Dimyristoylphosphatidylcholine	Ribbons
AmBisome	NexStar	Distearoylphosphatidylglycerol soy lecithin cholesterol	Small unilamellar vesicles
ABCD (Amphotec®)	Liposome Technology Inc.	Cholesteryl sulfate	Micelle

lipid rich tissues, is released in small amounts over long periods of time. The terminal half-life of amphotericin B is approximately 14 days. Administration of the drug may have to be held or the dose decreased in patients with worsening renal function, since renal failure is a major toxicity of amphotericin B.

Amphotericin B is indicated for the treatment of most life-threatening mycoses. Some fungi are inherently resistant, such as *Pseudallescheria boydii, Candida guillermondii, Candida krusei,* and *Candida lusitaniae.* Patients with severe, disseminated infection caused by the endemic fungi (e.g., *Blastomyces dermatitidis, Coccidioides immitis, Histoplasma capsulatum,* and *Paracoccidioides brasiliensis*) usually should receive amphotericin B initially. Azole therapy can be used once the patient has been stabilized.

Details on the use of amphotericin B for specific fungal infections are provided in the treatment section of previous chapters describing the individual mycoses.

Side Effects

Conventional amphotericin B (Fungizone) has many side effects (Table 12). The most important systemic toxicities are fever, chills, and rigors, which are associated with the infusion itself. The mechanism of these side effects may be related to the ability of amphotericin B to induce release of prostaglandins or tumor necrosis factor (TNF) from phagocytes. Thus, premedication with a prostaglandin inhibitor, such as ibuprofen, may be beneficial. Since nonsteroidal anti-inflammatory agents also have platelet-inhibiting properties, they may be relatively contraindicated in patients with thrombocytopenia. Whether decreasing infusion duration ameliorates these reactions is controversial.

Traditionally, amphotericin B has been infused over a 4- to 6-hour period, but in patients with normal renal function, infusions as short as

TABLE 12. *Side Effects of Amphotericin B*

Side Effect	Frequency	Comments
Systemic	>70%	Often controlled by hydrocortisone 25 mg; acetaminophen 650 to 1,000 mg; diphenhydramine 50 mg; meperidine (for rigors) 50 mg iv. Ibuprofen 400 mg may also be useful.
Fever		Treat with acetaminophen or a nonsteroidal anti-inflammatory, if indicated.
Chills		
Rigors		Treat with meperidine 50 mg iv, if indicated
Nausea/vomiting		Symptomatic treatment, if indicated
Headache	Rare	
Arthralgias	Rare	
Renal	>80%	Potentiated by dehydration and salt depletion; may ameliorate by saline loading (see text)
Increased BUN/Cr		
Decreased K^+, Mg^{+2}		Replace cations as needed, po or iv
Hepatic	Rare	Discontinue amphotericin N if values increase >3× upper limit of normal
Increased transaminases		
Increased alkaline phosphatase		
Hematologic		
Normocytic normochromic anemia	>50%	Due to decreased erythropoietin secretion
Leukopenia	Rare	
Thrombocytopenia	Rare	
Miscellaneous		
Cardiovascular		
Arrythmia	Rare	Likely secondary to elevated K^+; avoid rapid infusions (<2 h) in patients with renal insufficiency

45 minutes have been used without problems. A reasonable approach would be to infuse the drug over a 1- to 2-hour period. The problem with more rapid infusions in patients with renal insufficiency is that amphotericin B causes an increase in serum potassium (leakage from the intracellular spaces), and in renal failure, the kidney cannot excrete K^+ fast enough to prevent potentially toxic concentrations from developing in the blood.

The major organ specific toxicity of amphotericin B is on the kidney. Renal toxicity is due to direct effects of amphotericin B on renal blood flow, which is decreased, and on tubule function. As a result, not only does renal insufficiency develop in at least 80% of patients, loss of potassium and magnesium occurs, sometimes at a rapid rate, making monitoring of these ions essential. Most patients will sustain elevations of serum creatinine to about 3 mg/dl, and changes in dosage of amphotericin B are rarely required unless the serum creatinine increases above this empirically derived plateau. In such cases, either holding the dose until renal function stabilizes or decreasing the dose should be considered. Finally, renal tubular acidosis can occur. All of the renal effects of amphotericin B are potentiated by salt depletion and concomitant use of other nephrotoxic drugs (e.g., cyclosporine, aminoglycosides, pentamidine). If the patient can tolerate salt loading, some authorities recommend an infusion of normal saline, 500 ml prior to and 500 ml following, the infusion of amphotericin B. Unfortunately, patients with diminished cardiac reserve often cannot handle this amount of sodium. Permanent renal damage is uncommon with total cumulative amphotericin B doses of less than 4 g.

Less commonly, elevations of transaminases or alkaline phosphatase occur with conventional amphotericin B. Elevations in liver function tests more commonly are seen with liposomal preparations of amphotericin B and are of uncertain clinical significance.

The major effect of amphotericin B on the blood is the development of anemia. This is typically normocytic and normochromic, reversible, and due to inhibition of erythropoietin synthesis by amphotericin B. Leukopenia occurs rarely, and inhibition of phagocyte function may occur, but the clinical implications of this are unknown.

Miscellaneous toxicities reported with amphotericin B are indicated in Table 12. Most patients receive amphotericin B through central intravenous catheters. However, should peripheral veins be used, thrombophlebitis commonly occurs. To minimize this effect, addition of heparin (e.g., 1,000 U) to the amphotericin B bottle, slowing the infusion rate to 4 to 6 hours, rotation of use of peripheral veins, application of warm packs to the intravenous site, and the use of inline filters have all been suggested.

Drug Interactions

Conventional amphotericin B cannot be reconstituted in saline and must be reconstituted in 5% dextrose. Heparin and hydrocortisone can be added to the infusion mixture, but other drugs should not be mixed with amphotericin B to avoid precipitation of the antifungal agent.

Enhanced nephrotoxicity can be seen with concomitant use of amphotericin B and cyclosporine. Similarly, the nephrotoxicity of aminoglycosides is often increased when amphotericin B is also administered.

Acute pulmonary decompensation has been reported in most, but not all, publications examining an interaction between amphotericin B and white blood cell transfusion. Presumably, amphotericin B causes aggregation of the transfused leukocytes, which then become sequestered in the lungs. A picture compatible with adult respiratory distress syndrome then ensues. Given the low frequency of such transfusions, this remains more a theoretical concern.

Several different liposomal and lipid-associated formulations of amphotericin B have been introduced into clinical investigation and two have been approved for use. Amphotericin B Lipid Complex (ABLC, Ablecet) was approved for use in late 1995 and Amphotericin B Colloidal Dispersion (ABCD) was approved by the FDA in late 1996. It is a formulation in which the amphotericin B is associated with the lipid component, but true liposomes are not formed. AmBisome should become available for clinical use in the USA by the end of 1997.

NYSTATIN

Nystatin is a polyene that is currently available only as a topical agent (Fig. 11). Nystatin is used for the treatment of mucosal candidiasis, and is available as lozenges, suspension, or vaginal suppositories. Studies of intravenously injected liposomal nystatin are underway to assess its safety and efficacy in the treatment of invasive candidiasis and other mycoses. Topical nystatin is known to have a bitter taste, and usually is given four to five times daily to effect a response.

17

The Azoles: Ketoconazole, Fluconazole, Itraconazole, and Miconazole

The azole antifungals represent a diverse group of compounds administered by topical, oral, and intravenous routes. They act by inhibiting the synthesis of ergosterol, thereby destabilizing the fungal cell membrane. They are divided on the basis of chemical structure into imidazoles (clotrimazole, miconazole, and ketoconazole) and triazoles (fluconazole and itraconazole).

A comparison of the available oral azole antifungals is presented in Table 13 and a summary of their spectra of activity can be found in Table 14.

TABLE 13. *Important Pharmacologic Parameters for Oral Azoles*

Parameter	Ketoconazole	Fluconazole	Itraconazole
Route of administration	po	po, iv	po
Formulation	Tablet	Tablet, solution (for iv use)	Capsule
Water solubility	Low	Yes	Very low
Stomach acid required for optimal absorption	Yes	No	Yes
Food in stomach required for optimal absorption	No	No	Yes
Protein binding	99%	10%	99%
Half-life ($t_{1/2}$)	9 hours	24 hours	15 to 42 hours
Clearance	liver	Kidney	Liver
Metabolism	Extensive (>90%)	Minimal (<10%)	Extensive (>70%)
Urine concentrations	Low	High	Very low
CSF concentrations	Low	High	Very low

TABLE 14. *Utility of Oral Azoles Against Different Fungal Pathogens*

Fungus	Ketoconazole	Fluconazole	Itraconazole
Aspergillus species	0	0	++++
Candida albicans	Invasive disease 0; mucosal disease ++	Invasive disease ++++; mucosal disease ++++	Invasive disease ++++; mucosal disease ++ or ++++ (especially fluconazole-resistant isolates)
Candida non-*albiacans* species (*parapsilosis, tropicalis*)	Invasive disease +; mucosal disease ++	Invasive disease ++ or ++++; mucosal disease ++++	Invasive disease ++; mucosal disease ++ or ++++ (especially fluconazole-resistant isolates)
Candida (Torulopsis) glabrata	Invasive disease 0; mucosal disease +	Invasive disease ++ or ++++; mucosal disease ++++	Invasive disease ++; mucosal disease ++ or ++++ (especially fluconazole-resistant isolates)
Agents of Mucormycosis	0	0	0
Pseudallescheria boydii	++	++	++++
Blastomyces dermatitidis	++	+	++++
Coccidioides immitis, nonmeningeal	++	++++	++
Coccidioides immitis, meningeal	+	++++	++
Histoplasma capsulatum	++	+	++++
Paracoccidioides brasilensis	++	+	++++
Sporothrix schenkii	+	+	++++

++++ = preferred; ++ = active, but second-line agent; + = active but clinical failures common; 0 = do not use.

KETOCONAZOLE

Ketoconazole is an imidazole derivative (Fig. 12) and is available as a 200-mg tablet. (Nizoral®). The usual dose is 200 to 400 mg, given once daily. Larger doses can be given but are frequently complicated by gastrointestinal upset, with nausea and vomiting. As discussed below, higher doses, especially when given in divided doses three to four times per day, are associated with significant endocrinologic effects. Large doses of ketoconazole have been used for a variety of nonantifungal indications (e.g., prostate cancer and suppression of corticosteroid synthesis in patients with hyperproduction of these steroids).

Absorption is erratic, but can be maximized by maintaining stomach acid secretion and by ingesting the drug with a carbonated beverage, such as seltzer or cola. Dissolution of the tablets is more complete in carbonated soft drinks than in orange juice, which is recommended in the package insert.

Following oral administration of 200 mg, peak serum concentrations of 2 to 4 μg/ml are usually obtained. Ketoconazole is highly protein-bound and penetration of the drug into cerebrospinal fluid, saliva, and urine is extremely poor. Of some clinical import, there is no correlation between serum concentration and clinical outcome.

The elimination half-life of ketoconazole is about nine hours. It is extensively metabolized and undergoes an enterohepatic circulation. Less than 1% of the biologically active drug is excreted into the urine. Dosage adjustment is unnecessary in patients with renal failure. Minimal amounts of ketoconazole are removed by hemodialysis or peritoneal dialysis.

Indications

Ketoconazole has found most use in the treatment of patients with non-life-threatening infection with one of the dimorphic fungi causing the endemic mycosis. Thus, the drug has been found to be useful in treating patients with blastomycosis, nonmeningeal coccidioidomycosis, histoplasmosis, and paracoccidioidomycosis. Mucosal candidiasis, including chronic mucocutaneous candidiasis is also amenable to treatment with ketoconazole.

Ketoconazole is not recommended for the treatment of sporotrichosis, cryptococcosis, chromoblastomycosis, or any of the fungal meninigitides.

KETOCONAZOLE:

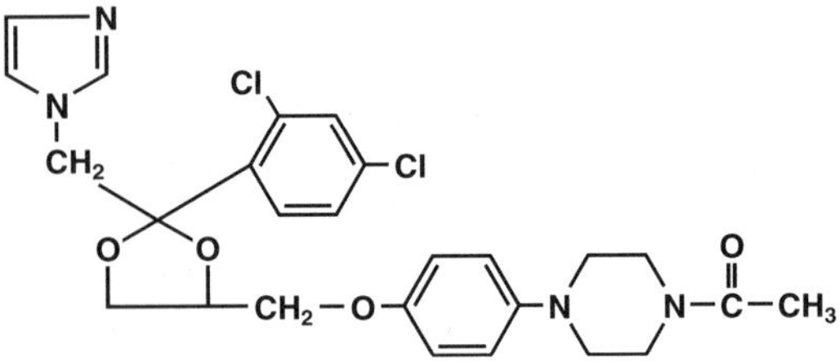

A

MICONAZOLE:

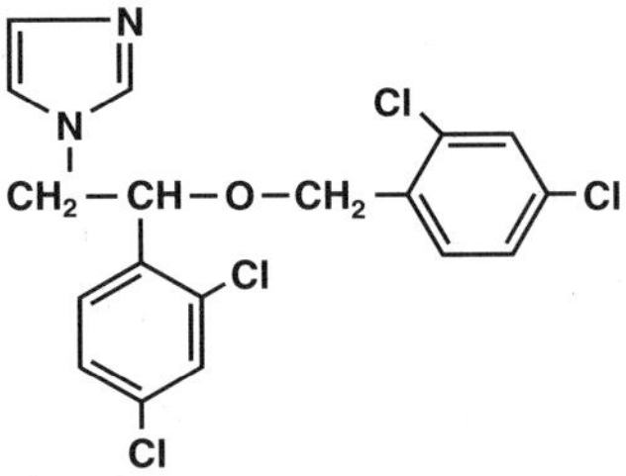

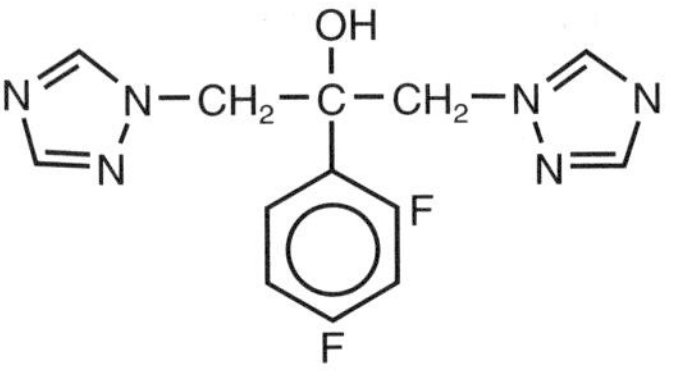

B

FLUCONAZOLE

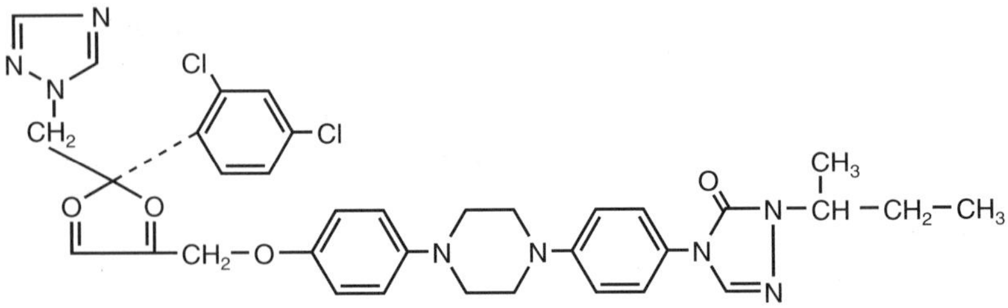

ITRACONAZOLE

FIG. 12. Structures of several important azole derivatives. **A:** Imidazole derivatives. **B:** Triazole derivatives.

Side Effects

The gastrointestinal tract is the site most commonly affected by ketoconazole. Increasing doses lead to increased nausea and vomiting, and over half of all patients taking more than 800 mg/day will exhibit this toxicity.

Hepatotoxicity of varying severity occurs and does not appear to be dose-related. Elevations of serum transaminases are seen in 2% to 8% of patients taking the drug. Progressive hepatitis ending in death can occur if a patient continues to take the drug in the face of continued worsening of the liver function tests. Progressive hepatitis of this sort occurs in approximately 1 in 10,000 patients.

In doses ≥ 400 mg/day, endocrine side effects are noted. Because ketoconazole inhibits mammalian cytochrome P450 enzymes, a variety of effects due to inhibition of androgenic steroids have been described and include impotence, oligospermia, decreased libido, and gynecomastia. Women may experience menstrual irregularities. At doses ≥ 800 mg/day, adrenal corticosteroid synthesis may be inhibited, but clinically evident adrenal insufficiency has rarely been documented.

Drug Interactions (Table 15)

Ketoconazole inhibits the metabolism of cyclosporine, thereby increasing serum cyclosporine concentrations. In fact, this interaction has been exploited to decrease the total daily dose of cyclosporine required, and thus the expense of this immunosuppressive agent. Concomitant administration of rifampin will result in enhanced metabolism of ketoconazole and lower blood concentrations of the antifungal agent. Concomitant use of ketoconazole with cisapride, astemizole, or terfenadine is contraindicated since there is an increased risk of cardiac arrhythmias, including torsade de pointes.

Antacids and H_2 blockers (e.g., cimetidine and ranitidine) decrease blood levels of ketoconazole by increasing stomach pH, and thereby decreasing the absorption of the drug.

ITRACONAZOLE

Itraconazole is a water-insoluble triazole derivative and is available as 100-mg capsules (Sporanox®). Suspensions for oral use and an intravenous preparation are undergoing clinical trials, but are not yet clini-

TABLE 15. *Drug Interactions With Azoles*

Interaction	Ketoconazole	Fluconazole	Itraconazole
Decreased azole blood concentration			
H_2 blockers, antacids	++++	0	++++
Didanosine (ddI)	++++	0	++++
Carbamazepine	++++	0	++++
Phenytoin	++++	0	++++
Rifampin	++++	++	++++
Increased blood concentration of other drugs			
Astemizole	++++	0	++++
Cyclosporine	++++	+	+
Cisapride	++++	0	++++
Digoxin	++++	++	++++
Phenytoin	++++	++	++++
Sulfonylurea	++++	0	++
Terfenadine	++++	0	++++
Theophylline	?	+	?
Warfarin	++	+	++

++++ = marked effect (clinically important); ++ = moderate effect (still clinically important); + = some effect (usually not clinically important); 0 = no effect.

cally available. The usual dose depends on the infection being treated, but 100 to 400 mg daily are used most commonly, with higher doses being split into two, e.g., 200 mg bid. Dosages exceeding 400 mg per day are associated with an increase in side effects (see below).

The absorption of itraconazole is erratic and is dependent on a low gastric pH and food in the stomach. Absorption may be further optimized by carbonated beverages. Following oral administration of 200 mg, peak serum concentrations of 4 to 6 μg/ml are obtained when measured by bioassay. Serum concentrations of the drug can be measured by bioassay or HPLC, with bioassay yielding higher values. This is due in part to the extensive metabolism of itraconazole and the production of an active hydroxylated metabolites, which is measured in the bioassay but not usually in the HPLC. In order to document that absorption is occurring, it is advisable to monitor serum concentrations. Steady state concentrations are achieved in about 2 weeks, when a loading dose is not used. The serum half-life is about 20 hours. Itraconazole is widely distributed throughout the body, but does not appear in CSF or urine to any appreciable degree. No dosage adjustment is needed in patients with renal insufficiency.

Side Effects

Itraconazole is tolerated much better than ketoconazole, and the need for discontinuation of the drug is unusual when dosages are ≤ 400 mg/day. The most common side effects are gastrointestinal, with nausea and vomiting occurring in about 10% of patients. Increases in triglycerides have been reported in 9%, hypokalemia in 6%, increases in transaminases in 5%, and skin rashes in 2% of patients. In doses <400 mg daily, endocrinologic side effects are distinctly unusual. However, some patients receiving 400 mg per day or more can present with an aldosterone-like effect and complain of peripheral edema and have hypertension and hypokalemia. Clinically evident hepatitis is rare.

Drug Interactions (Table 15)

Concomitant use of itraconazole with cisapride, astemizole, or terfenadine is contraindicated, because there is an increased risk of cardiac arrhythmias, including torsade de pointes.

FLUCONAZOLE

Fluconazole (Diflucan®) is a water-soluble triazole derivative. Fluconazole tablets are available in 50-, 100-, and 200-mg strengths, as well as 10 and 40 mg/ml oral suspensions in the United States. A special 150-mg tablet is also available for the single-dose treatment of *Candida* vaginitis. An intravenous formulation is also available in concentrations of 200 mg and 400 mg, in 100- and 200-ml suspensions, respectively.

A key feature of this drug is its high absorption from the gastrointestinal track, regardless of stomach acid or food content (bioavailability about 90%). In contrast to ketoconazole and itraconazole, most of the drug is not protein-bound and is excreted in active form in the urine. Because the primary route of excretion is in the urine, the dose should be decreased in patients with renal insufficiency (Table 16).

Children have more rapid clearance of fluconazole than do adults. Therefore, the comparisons of pediatric with adult doses of the drug are as follows:

Pediatric dose	Adult equivalent
3 mg/kg	100 mg
6 mg/kg	200 mg
12 mg/kg	400 mg

Side Effects

Side effects of fluconazole include nausea (2.5%), abdominal pain (1.7%), diarrhea (1.2%), and vomiting (1%). At doses less than 1,600 mg/day endocrinologic toxicity has not been noted. Transaminase elevations may occur, but clinically evident hepatitis is extremely rare. Skin rash has been rare, but an association of the use of fluconazole with the development of Stevens-Johnson syndrome has been reported. Patients who develop skin rashes, especially with the formation of vesicles, should stop taking fluconazole and be observed closely for progression of lesions.

Azoles are considered to be teratogenic, and birth defects following administration of fluconazole have been reported. Thus, suitable precautions should be taken to insure that women taking this drug are not pregnant.

Fluconazole is useful in the treatment of acute and suppressive therapy of cryptococcosis, superficial forms of candidiasis (such as thrush, esophagitis, and vaginitis), candidemia, candidal urinary tract infections, hepatosplenic candidiasis, and coccidioidomycosis (acute pulmonary and meningitis). Experience with its use in histoplasmosis and blastomycosis is limited, but doses of 400 mg and higher are likely to be needed based on early studies with the lower doses.

Fluconazole has no activity against *Aspergillus* spp. or the agents of mucormycosis, and should not be used for treating any form of these infections. Its role in the treatment of infections caused by *Pseudallescheria boydii* remains to be clarified, but the drug may be effective in this setting. Sporotrichosis is probably better treated with itraconazole.

TABLE 16. *Dosage Modification of Fluconazole in Patients With Renal Insufficiency*

Creatinine Clearance	% of Recommended Usual Dose
>50 ml/min	100
11–50 ml/min	50
Hemodialysis	100 (after each dialysis)

Fluconazole resistance has been identified in *Candida* species, primarily in AIDS patients with oropharyngeal candidiasis. One explanation for this development is that the drug has been used at low doses (50 to 100 mg daily) in patients with limited or no innate host immune system function. In this setting, clinical resistance has appeared; using standardized *in vitro* antifungal susceptibility testing methods, MICs to fluconazole have been noted to increase. MICs ≥ 64 μg/ml are usually associated with lack of clinical response to fluconazole doses of ≤ 800 mg/day in these patients. In contrast, similar *in vitro/in vivo* correlations have not been demonstrable in patients with invasive candidiasis and clinical or laboratory resistance has not been observed.

There are several mechanisms of azole resistance. Clinically, patients may be infected with heterogeneous populations of varying susceptibility to the drugs. With therapy, the susceptible population is initially eradicated and the more-resistant population grows to fill the ecological void. The resistant organisms may be inherently resistant to fluconazole (e.g., *C. krusei*) or resistance may develop during therapy. In this latter instance, several reasons can explain the decrease in susceptibility of the fungus. There may be an alteration in the target enzyme, cytochrome P450, so that the azole cannot bind to the enzyme, resulting in a lack of inhibition. Fungi exhibiting this feature usually demonstrate cross resistance to all azoles. Another potential explanation for this resistance is either decreased influx or increased efflux, so that intracellular concentrations of the drug are decreased. Finally, a general increase in the amount of cytochrome P450 in the cell can compensate for the inhibitory effects of the antifungal and ergosterol synthesis sufficient to maintain growth. Given the variety of mechanisms for azole resistance, cross resistance to all azoles is a real possibility; it should not be assumed that fluconazole-resistant strains will always be susceptible to other azoles, such as itraconazole.

Fluconazole has relatively fewer clinically important drug interactions than do the other available azole drugs (listed in Table 15).

MICONAZOLE

This imidazole derivative is available for intravenous and topical use only. Miconazole is rarely the antifungal drug of choice because of its relative narrow spectrum of activity, the need for intravenous dosing four times daily, and a unique set of side effects. Prior to the availability of the broader spectrum oral triazoles, miconazole was used for treating candidiasis, coccidioidomycosis, and pseudallescheriosis. In fact, the latter infection is probably the only current indication for the use of intravenous miconazole. Itraconazole, however, may replace miconazole as the drug of choice for treating infections caused by *P. boydii,* although data still are limited.

Side Effects

Side effects of intravenously administered miconazole include pruritus, headache, phlebitis, and hepatitis. Rouleaux formation of erythrocytes on peripheral blood smears is caused by the lipid vehicle used to suspend the drug. Miconazole should not be used in patients requiring cisapride, since interactions result in cardiac arrhythmias, including torsade de pointes.

MISCELLANEOUS AZOLES MARKETED IN THE U.S. FOR THE TREATMENT OF CANDIDA VAGINITIS

These drugs may be available as creams or suppositories and are for the topical treatment of Candida vaginitis only. Some are available over the counter, as well as by prescription. Course of therapy usually ranges from 3 to 7 days.

Butoconazole (FemStat)
Clotrimazole (Canesten, Clotrimaderm, Gyne-Lotrimin, FemCare, Mycelex, Myco-Gyne)
Miconazole (Monistat)
Terconazole (Terazol)
Tioconazole (Vagistat, Gyno-Trosyd)

Side Effects

The side effects of these agents are summarized in Table 17.

TABLE 17. *Side effects of azoles used for treating vaginal candidiasis*

Vaginal burning, itching, discharge
Hypersensitivity
Irritation of penis of sexual partner
Abdominal pain

AZOLES ON THE HORIZON

Several new azole derivatives are in various phases of preclinical drug development. It is not known which, if any, of these will complete the drug-evaluation process and be licensed for clinical use. However, it is useful to be aware that these new compounds may become available over the next few years.

Voriconazole (Pfizer Pharmaceuticals) is a broad-spectrum triazole derivative and has been studied in patients in Europe, with studies to begin in the United States in early 1997. The drug has advantages over fluconazole, in that its spectrum of activity includes *Aspergillus* species and fluconazole-resistant yeasts. Oral and intravenous formulations should be available.

SCH 56592 (Schering-Plough Corp.) is a broad-spectrum triazole derivative with activity against many different yeasts and molds, including fluconazole-resistant yeasts and *Aspergillus* spp. The drug has a long half-life, and once-daily (or less frequent) dosing may be possible.

18

Flucytosine

Flucytosine (Ancoban®) was introduced into clinical practice in the 1970s, but has not proved to be useful as a single-agent therapy. However, in combination with amphotericin B or the oral triazoles, improved response to the antifungal regimen can be expected. Flucytosine (5-fluorocytosine), a pyrimidine derivative (Fig. 13), acts by inhibiting protein synthesis by blocking steps in the synthesis of DNA and RNA. Single-agent therapy has not been useful since many fungi are resistant or develop resistance rapidly to this drug.

Flucytosine is water soluble and is given orally as a capsule, since about 80% to 90% of the administered dose is absorbed from the gastrointestinal tract. Minimal amounts of the drug are protein-bound. The half-life is approximately 4 hours. Excretion is through the kidneys, with 90% being excreted unchanged in the urine. Therefore, dose reduction is important in patients with renal failure (Table 18). An intravenous formulation of flucytosine is unavailable.

Side effects of flucytosine are largely dose-related. The major toxicity occurring in 5% to 10% of patients are nausea, vomiting, and diarrhea. Elevations of hepatic transaminases occur with a similar frequency. Some patients complain of headache or light-headedness. Bone marrow suppression is the most serious flucytosine-related toxicity, especially affecting white blood cell and platelet counts. It is thought that conversion of flucytosine to 5-fluorouracil in the intestinal tract is responsible for the majority of these toxicities.

Doses are typically administered four times daily. Recent studies suggest that doses of 75 to 100 mg/kg/day are appropriate in most patients with normal renal function in order to maintain serum concentrations in the range of 50 to 75 mg/ml. It is important to keep serum concentrations of flucytosine below 100 mg/ml to avoid the dose-related toxicities.

Flucytosine is recommended in combination with amphotericin B in the treatment of cryptococcal meningitis. However, the original studies

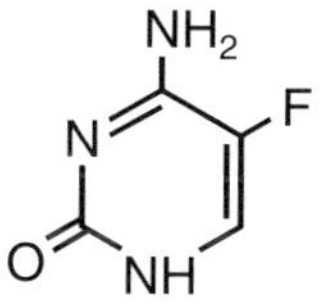

Flucytosine

FIG. 13. Structure of flucytosine.

with this combination therapy added the flucytosine in order to reduce the dose of amphotericin B necessary, in order to minimize the toxicity related to that drug. Thus, many experts now consider the doses of amphotericin B used in those studies (0.3. mg/kg/day) too low and would prefer to use doses of approximately 0.7 mg/kg/day. Amphotericin B-related renal insufficiency is extremely common at this dose, and, thus, complicates proper dosing of the flucytosine.

In combination with fluconazole (400 to 800 mg/day), improved response rates have been seen in patients with cryptococcal meningitis, and this form of therapy can be considered on a case-by-case basis.

Finally, some authorities recommend the addition of flucytosine to amphotericin B in the treatment of patients with invasive aspergillosis. However, a role for flucytosine in improving response rates has not been demonstrated, and since many of these patients have neutropenia, the flucytosine-related toxicity on bone marrow may further complicate the use of the drug in this setting.

Drug Interactions

Since flucytosine is most often given in combination with amphotericin B, it is the most important interaction to consider with this drug. Since renal function very frequently deteriorates when a patient receives

TABLE 18. *Dosage Recommendations for Flucytosine*

Creatinine clearance (ml/min)	Dosing interval (hr)
>40	6
20–40	12
10–20	24

amphotericin B, increases in serum concentrations of flucytosine often occur subsequently, increasing the risk of toxicity. Thus, it is important to measure serum concentrations of flucytosine at least weekly and more frequently if renal function is changing.

In addition, any drug that causes neutropenia or other bone marrow suppression, such as chemotherapeutic agents, can have additive detrimental effects on the bone marrow when administered with flucytosine.

19

Investigational Antifungal Drugs

The only currently available clinically effective antifungals for the treatment of invasive mycoses have targeted the fungal cell membrane. Thus, polyenes (which bind to fungal cell membrane sterols) and azoles (which inhibit ergosterol synthesis leading to destabilization of the fungal cell membrane) have been the only antifungal agents satisfactory for widespread clinical use. Flucytosine, an inhibitor of DNA synthesis, has also been available for clinical use, but the rapid development of resistance and narrow spectrum of activity have limited its utility.

Although current antifungals exploit a limited number of fungal targets, numerous examples of other fungal targets may yield specific antifungal drugs. For example, the fungal cell wall can be attacked by compounds directed toward synthesis of glucan, chitin, or mannan. Enzymes responsible for the synthesis of DNA or RNA, such as polymerases, may also be inhibited by drugs exhibiting differential specificity toward the fungal rather than the human enzyme. A few of these newer drugs currently under development are briefly reviewed below.

ALLYLAMINES

These compounds are reversible, noncompetitive inhibitors of squalene epoxidase, a key enzyme in the synthetic pathway for ergosterol. Accumulation of squalene and depletion of ergosterol results in loss of critical membrane functions. Naftifine and terbinafine are in clinical use and are available for topical administration. Terbinafine, as an oral agent, is also being investigated for its use in the treatment of invasive mycoses.

MORPHOLINES

These synthetic agents, like the allylamines, inhibit ergosterol synthesis by inhibiting two additional enzymes involved in the complex ergosterol biosynthetic pathway. Amorolfine is the only compound in this class currently available and it is used as a topical agent only. Systemic administration of these drugs is not possible since the drugs manifest unacceptable toxicity.

ECHINOCANDINS AND PNEUMOCANDINS

These molecules are noncompetitive inhibitors of 1,3-β-glucan synthetase, an enzyme critical in the synthesis of glucan, large polymers comprising an important fraction of the fungal cell wall. Cilofungin, the first echinocandin used in humans, progressed through phase II trials. However, toxicity associated with the polyethylene glycol vehicle needed to deliver the highly hydrophobic drug intravenously, halted further clinical development of this compound. More recently, water-soluble derivatives with antifungal and anti-*Pneumocystis* activity have been identified and synthesized, and due to activity against the latter organism, these compounds are referred to as pneumocandins.

POLYOXINS AND NIKKOMYCINS

These drugs are under investigation, but have not yet become clinically useful. They inhibit the synthesis of chitin, a critical component of the fungal cell wall that is not part of the mammalian cell. The nikkomycins and polyoxins are the prototypic members of this class of drugs. In order to be effective, these agents require transport into the fungal cell via a peptide permease. However, uptake into the fungal cell in an infected host is poor, resulting in de facto resistance to the drug. Thus, derivatives of these agents that bypass the peptide transporter are being sought as a potential means to overcome may be one answer to the problem of innate resistance to this group of antifungal drugs.

BENANOMICINS AND PRADIMICINS

These compounds are active following interactions with mannoproteins, which are important constituents of the fungal cell. Once bound to the fungal cell, these compounds destabilize the fungal cell membrane by unknown mechanisms. They have a broad spectrum of activity and appear to have low toxicity. The development of suitable derivatives of the parent compounds is underway.

APPENDICES

Appendix 1

Simple Classification of Medically Important Fungi

"Opportunistic" Fungi
Alternaria
Aspergillus sp.
Candida sp.
Fusarium sp.
Pseudallescheria boydii (*Scedosporium* spp.)
Trichosporon beigelii

"Endemic" Fungi (also called the Dimorphic Fungi)
Blastomyces dermatitidis
Coccidioides immitis
Histoplasma capsulatum
Paracoccidioides brasiliensis
*Sporothrix schenkii**

**Sporothrix schenkii* is not geographically restricted as are the other dimorphic fungal pathogens, so it is technically not a cause of an "endemic mycosis."

Appendix 2

Names of Fungi and Mycoses and Synonyms

Currently Accepted Name	Synonym
Acremonium	*Cephalosporium*
Candida albicans	*Monilia albicans*
Cladosporium bantianum	*Cladosporium trichoides*
Conidiobolus coronatus	*Entomophthora coronata*
Exophiala jeanselmei	*Phialophora jeanselmei*
Exophiala werneckii	*Cladosporium werneckii*
Fonsecaea compacta	*Phialophora compacta, Rhioncladiella compacta*
Fonsecaea pedrosoi	*Phialophora pedrosoi, Rhinocladiella pedrosoi*
Histoplasma capsulatum var. *duboisii*	*Histoplasma duboisii*
Malassezia furfur	*Pityrosporum orbiculare, Pityrosporum ovale*
Mucormycosis	Zygomycosis
Pseudallescheria boydii	*Allescheria boydii, Petriellidium boydii*
Rhizomucor pusillus	*Mucor pusillus*
Scedosporium apiospermum	*Monosporium apiospermum*
Sporothrix schenckii	*Sporotrichum schenckii*
Wangiella dermatitidis	*Exophiala dermatitidis, Phialophora dermatitidis, Fonsecaea dermatitidis*

Appendix 3

Fungi Recovered From Soil

Aspergillus species
*Coccidioides immitis**
Cryptococcus neoformans
Fusarium spp.
*Histoplasma capsulatum**
Phialophora spp.
Pseudallescheria boydii (*Scedosporium apiospermum*)
Sporothrix schenkii

*In the appropriate endemic area

Appendix 4

Fungal Infections Caused by Fungi That Are Inhaled

Caused by "Opportunistic" Fungi
Aspergillosis
Cryptococcosis
Mucormycosis
Pseudallescheriosis

Caused by Endemic Mycoses
Blastomycosis
Coccidioidomycosis
Histoplasmosis
Paracoccidioidomycosis

Appendix 5

Fungal Infections Caused by Fungi Which Usually Enter the Body Through Nonpulmonary Routes

Candidiasis
Sporotrichosis
Fusariosis
Phaeohyphomycosis (dematiacious fungal infections)

Appendix 6

Common Fungal Infections Acquired in the Hospital

Disease	Source
Aspergillosis	Airborne; possibly construction work, potted plants
Candidiasis	Usually endogenous source (e.g., patient's own gastrointestinal tract), intravenous catheters, Foley catheters, fomites, hands of personnel

Appendix 7

Fungal Pathogens in Cardiology*

Fungi	Usual Manifestations
Common	
Candida species	Endocarditis; myocarditis; pericarditis
Aspergillus species	Endocarditis; myocarditis; pericarditis
Rare	
Blastomyces dermatitidis	Myocarditis; pericarditis
Coccidioides immitis	Myocarditis; pericarditis
Cryptococcus neoformans	Myocarditis; pericarditis
Histoplasma capsulatum	Myocarditis; pericarditis
Trichosporon beigelii	Myocarditis; pericarditis
Pseudallescheria boydii	Myocarditis; pericarditis

*Most common manifestation is endocarditis, but rare cases of myocarditis, especially in patients with disseminated infections have been reported.

Appendix 8

Fungal Pathogens in Dermatology

Fungi	Usual Manifestations
Candida species	Primary cutaneous rashes; skin lesions secondary to invasive disease
Aspergillus species	Skin lesions secondary to invasive disease from dissemination or direct implantation
Fusarium species	Skin lesions secondary to dissemination
Agents of mucormycosis	Skin lesions secondary to dissemination or primary cutaneous infection secondary to direct inoculation
Dimorphic fungi	
Blastomyces dermatitidis	Skin lesions secondary to dissemination; direct implantation (very rare)
Coccidioides immitis	Skin lesions secondary to dissemination; direct implantation (very rare)
Histoplasma capsulatum	Skin lesions secondary to dissemination; direct implantation (very rare)
Paracoccidioides brasiliensis	Skin lesions secondary to dissemination; direct implantation (very rare)
Sporothrix schenkii	Skin lesions secondary to direct implantation
Penicillium marnefei	Skin lesions secondary to dissemination; direct implantation (very rare)
Dermatophytes (not covered in this book)	Primary superficial skin involvement

Appendix 9

Fungal Pathogens in Gastroenterology

Fungus	Usual Manifestations
Candida spp.	Oropharyngeal thrush; esophagitis
Cryptococcus neoformans	Intestines
Blastomyces dermatitidis	Intestines
Coccidioides immitis	Intestines
Histoplasma capsulatum	Oral mucosa; intestines
Paracoccidioides brasiliensis	Oral mucosa; intestines
Sporothrix schenkii	Intestines
Mucorales	Intestines

Appendix 10

Fungal Pathogens in Neurology/Neurosurgery

Fungus	Usual Manifestations*
Common	
Cryptococcus neoformans	Meningitis > mass lesions
Coccidioides immitis	Meningitis > mass lesions
Histoplasma capsulatum	Meningitis > mass lesions
Uncommon	
Aspergillus spp.	Mass lesions > meningitis
Blastomyces dermatitidis	Meningitis > mass lesions
Candida spp.	Meningitis > mass lesions
Mucorales	Mass lesions > meningitis
Paracoccidioides brasiliensis	Meningitis > mass lesions
Sporothrix schenkii	Meningitis > mass lesions
Dematiacious (pigmented) fungi	Mass lesions > meningitis

*Relative frequencies of the presentations are given when known.

Appendix 11

Fungal Pathogens in OB/GYN

- *Candida* species
  - *C. albicans*
  - *C. tropicalis*
  - *C. parapsilosis*
  - *C. glabrata (Torulopsis glabrata)*
- *Aspergillus* spp. (rare)

Appendix 12

Fungal Pathogens in Ophthalmology

Keratitis
Fusarium spp.
Aspergillus spp.
Candida spp.
Pseudallescheria boydii
Alternaria
Penicillium
Curvularia
Dematiaceous fungi

Endophthalmitis
Candida
Aspergillus
Cryptococcus neoformans
Mucorales
Fusarium spp.
Pseudallescheria boydii
Trichosporon spp.
Blastomyces dermatitidis
Coccidioides immitis
Histoplasma capsulatum
Sporothrix schenkii

Appendix 13

Fungal Pathogens in Orthopedics

Fungus	Usual Manifestations*
Endemic fungi	
Blastomyces dermatitidis	Osteomyelitis > septic arthritis
Coccidioides immitis	Osteomyelitis = septic arthritis
Histoplasma capsulatum	Osteomyelitis = septic arthritis (both rare)
Paracoccidioides brasiliensis	Osteomyelitis (rare)
Opportunistic fungi	
Candida spp.	Osteomyelitis; septic arthritis (both rare)
Cryptococcus neoformans	Osteomyelitis > septic arthritis
Others	
Sporothrix schenkii	Septic arthritis; osteomyelitis (both rare)

*Relative frequencies of the presentations are given when known

Appendix 14

Fungal Pathogens in Otolaryngology

Fungus	Usual Manifestations
Common	
Aspergillus spp.	Otitis externa, malignant otitis externa, sinusitis (may be indistinguishable from certain presentations of mucormycosis
Candida spp.	Thrush, otitis externa, laryngitis (rare)
Mucorales	Sinusitis, rhinocerebral mucormycosis
Alternaria	Sinusitis (nasal polyps, allergic sinusitis, rarely invasive sinusitis)
Fusarium	Sinusitis
Uncommon	
Rhinosporidium	Nasal polyps and masses
Histoplasma capsulatum	Mucosal lesions
Paracoccidioides brasiliensis	Mucosal lesions

Appendix 15

Fungal Pathogens in Pulmonary Medicine

Fungi	Usual Manifestations
Aspergillus spp.	Pneumonia; tracheobronchitis; upper airway infection
Agents of mucormycosis	Upper airway infection; pneumonia
Dimorphic fungi	
Blastomyces dermatitidis	Pneumonia; disseminated infection
Coccidioides immitis	Pneumonia; disseminated infection
Histoplasma capsulatum	Pneumonia; disseminated infection
Paracoccidioides brasiliensis	Pneumonia; disseminated infection
Fusarium and other molds	Pneumonia; disseminated infection

Appendix 16

Fungal Pathogens in Urology

Fungi	Usual Manifestations
Candida spp.	Cystitis; pyelonephritis prostatitis; balanitis
Cryptococcus neoformans	Prostatitis; pyelonephritis
Trichosporon spp.	Cystitis; prostatitis
Aspergillus spp.	Pyelonephritis
Blastomyces dermatitidis	Prostatitis
Histoplasma capsulatum	Balanitis; penile lesions; pyelonephritis; prostatitis
Coccidioides immitis	Pyelonephritis

Appendix 17

Other Medically Important Fungi

Group/Disease	Examples	Clues to Diagnosis
Dematiaceous fungi usually dermal (pigmented fungi)	*Cladosporium, Fonsecaea, Exophiala, Alternaria*	Infection, occ. brain abscess; dark hyphae seen in tissue section, without special stains
Lobomycosis	*Loboa loboi*	Patients from South America
Protothecosis	*Prototheca wickerhamii, P. zopfi*	Algae, round structures (endospores) in cartwheel arrangement
Rhinosporidiosis	*Rhinosporidium seeberi*	Very large round structures, usually recovered from nasal mucosa or conjunctiva
Piedra	*Trichosporon, Piedraia*	Hair infections
Dermatophytes		Cutaneous and hair infections

For information concerning these mycoses, the reader is advised to consult one of the mycology textbooks or general Infectious Diseases textbooks listed in the Reference section of this book.

Appendix 18

Summary of Treatment Recommendations for Fungal Infections*

Disease	First-Line Therapy	Alternative Therapy	Comments
Aspergillosis	Amphotericin B	Itraconazole	Some may add rifampin to amphotericin B; use of amphotericin B with itraconazole or ketoconazole is probably antagonistic; however, initial therapy with amphotericin B followed by itraconazole seems to be clinically safe.
Blastomycosis	Itraconazole	Amphotericin B; fluconazole	
Candidiasis	Fluconazole	Amphotericin B, itraconazole	Combinations of fluconazole with amphotericin B may be useful.
Coccidioidomycosis	Itraconazole	Amphotericin B, fluconazole, ketoconazole	
Cryptococcosis	Amphotericin B ± Flucytosine	Fluconazole ± flucytosine, itraconazole	
Fusariosis	Amphotericin B	Fluconazole	
Histoplasmosis	Itraconazole	Amphotericin B	
Mucormycosis	Amphotericin B	None	
Pseudallescheriosis	Itraconazole	Miconazole; ketoconazole; fluconazole	
Sporotrichosis	Itraconazole	Amphotericin B, fluconazole	

*These are general guidelines. **See text** for more specific information.

In general, patients acutely ill with life-threatening mycosis should be treated with amphotericin B and azole therapy can follow once the patient's condition is stabilized.

Appendix 19

Dose Modifications of Antifungal Drugs in Renal Failure and Dialysis

Drug	Creatinine Clearance	Dose
Amphotericin B		No change; may want to hold dose or decrease by ± 50% when creatinine reaches 3 mg/dl **(see text)**
Fluconazole	>50 ml/min	100% of usual dose
	11–50 ml/min	50% of usual dose
	Hemodialysis	100% after each dialysis
Itraconazole		No change
Ketoconazole		No change
Miconazole		No change

Appendix 20

Laboratories Specializing in Clinical Testing for Fungal Diseases

Director	Laboratory	Comments
Leo Kaufman, Ph.D.	Centers for Disease Control, Mycotic Diseases Branch, Building 5, Room B13-G11, Atlanta, GA 30333	Fungal identification (send isolates to attention of Dr. Arvind Padhye)
Michael Pfaller, Ph.D.	Department of Pathology, University of Iowa College of Medicine, 273 MRC, Iowa City, Iowa 52242, phone: 319-335-8170, fax: 319-335-8348, email: michael-pfaller@uiowa.edu	Antifungal susceptibility testing; antifungal drug levels
Demosthenes Pappagianis, M.D., Ph.D.	University of California at Davis, School of Medicine, Department of Microbiology, and Immunology, Davis, Davis, CA 95616, phone: 916-752-3391, fax: 916-752-8692	Serologic testing for coccidioidomycosis
Michael Rinaldi, Ph.D.	Fungus Testing Laboratory, University of Texas, Health Sciences Center, 7703 Floyd Curl Drive, San Antonio, Texas 78284, phone: 210-567-4132, fax: 210-567-6729, email: rinaldi@uthscsa.edu	Fungal identification; antifungal susceptibility testing; antifungal drug levels
Alan M. Sugar, M.D.	Clinical Mycology Center, Boston Medical Center, 88 East Newton Street, Boston, Massachusetts 02118, phone: 617-638-7905, fax: 617-638-8070, email: asugar@med-med1.bu.edu	Antifungal susceptibility testing; antifungal drug levels

(continued on next page)

Appendix 20 (cont.)

Director	Laboratory	Comments
David A. Stevens, M.D.	Institute for Medical Research, 751 Basom Avenue, San Jose, California 95030, phone: 408-885-4313, fax: 408-885-4306, email: stevens@leland.stanford.edu	Antifungal, susceptibility testing; antifungal drug levels
L. Joseph Wheat, M.D.	Histoplasmosis Reference Laboratory, 1001 West 10th Street, OPW 430, Indianapolis, In 46202, phone:800-447-8634, fax: 317-630-2515, email: histodgn@indyunix.iupui.edu	Histoplasmosis antigen testing, itraconazole levels

Appendix 21

Key Terms Helpful in MedLine Searches

Diseases
Aspergillosis *(Aspergillus)*
Blastomycosis *(Blastomyces dermatitidis)*
Candidiasis *(Candida,* thrush, esophagitis)
Coccidioidomycosis *(Coccidioides immitis,* meningitis and coccidioidal)
Fusariosis *(Fusarium)*
Histoplasmosis *(Histoplasma capsulatum)*
Paracoccidioidomycosis *(Paracoccidioides brasiliensis)*
Pseudallescheriosis *(Pseudallescheria Petrellidium, Allescheria)*
Scedosporium
Sporotrichosis *(Sporothrix schenkii)*
Mucormycosis *(Cunninghamella, Rhizopus, Mucor,* Zygomycosis, also cite other specific genera)
Therapy
Antifungal
Polyene
Amphotericin
Nystatin
Azole
Fluconazole
Itraconazole
Ketoconazole
Miconazole
Allylamine
Naftifine
Terbinafine
Pneumocandin
Echinocandin
Cilofungin
Miscellaneous
Immunocompromised host, fungal infection
Mycosis
Fungal infection, fungal disease
Fungus, fungi

References

The field of medical mycology is rapidly advancing. New fungi routinely are being implicated as the cause of disease, and new formal mycological studies are being conducted and reported daily. Advances in diagnostic methodologies also are being made. Given the ease with which the world literature can be reviewed by electronic means, we have elected to provide here just a few of the standard helpful resources. We recommend that the reader obtain the most-up-to-date literature sources through these modern means of information retrieval.

STANDARD TEXT SOURCES

General

Fungal disease chapters in basic medicine and surgery textbooks are a good place to start when trying to answer clinical questions. There is also excellent fungal disease coverage in the following infectious diseases textbooks:

Gorbach SL, Bartlett JG, Blacklow NR: *Infectious Diseases.* WB Saunders, Philadelphia, 1996.
Hoeprich PD, Jordan MC, Ronald AR: *Infectious Diseases. A Treatise of Infectious Diseases,* Lippincott-Raven Publishers, New York, 1994.
Mandell GL, Bennett JE, Dolin R: *Principles and Practice of Infectious Diseases.* Churchill Livingstone, New York, 1995.

Specialty Textbooks

Bodey GP: *Candidiasis: Pathogenesis, Diagnosis, and Treatment.* Raven Press, New York, 1993.
Kibbler CC, Mackenzie DWR, Odds FC: *Principles and Practice of Clinical Mycology.* John Wiley and Sons, New York, 1996.
Kwon-Chung KJ, Bennet JE: *Medical Mycology.* Lea and Febiger, Philadelphia, 1992.
Meunier F: *Bailliere's Clinical Infectious Diseases: Invasive Fungal Infections in Cancer Patients.* Bailliere Tindall, London, 1995.
Rippon JW: *Medical Mycology: The Pathogenic Fungi and the Pathogenic Actinomycetes.* WB Saunders Company, Philadelphia, 1988.
Sarosi GA, Davies SF: *Fungal Diseases of the Lung.* Raven Press, New York, 1993.

Useful Journals

Fungal diseases are reported in journals of every medical and surgical specialty. These are typically case reports, reviews, or reports of therapy in varying numbers of patients with specific mycoses. Listed here are some of the more important specialty journals that provide clinical and basic information on fungi of medical interest.

Mycology
Journal of Medical and Veterinary Mycology (formerly Sabouraudia)
Mycopathologia
Mycoses

Infectious Diseases
Antimicrobial Agents and Chemotherapy
Clinical Infectious Diseases
Diagnostic Microbiology and Infectious Disease
Journal of Clinical Microbiology
Journal of Infectious Diseases

Subject Index

WC 450 S947 1997

Sugar, Alan M

Practical guide to
medically important fungi
and the deasease...

DEMCO